Dress and Society

Contributions from Archaeology

edited by
Toby F. Martin and Rosie Weetch

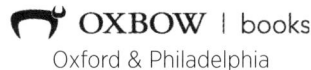

OXBOW | books
Oxford & Philadelphia

Published in the United Kingdom in 2017 by
OXBOW BOOKS
The Old Music Hall, 106–108 Cowley Road, Oxford OX4 1JE, UK

and in the United States by
OXBOW BOOKS
1950 Lawrence Road, Havertown, PA 19083

© Oxbow Books and the individual contributors 2017

Paperback Edition: ISBN 978-1-78570-315-7
Digital Edition: ISBN 978-1-78570-316-4 (epub)

A CIP record for this book is available from the British Library

Library of Congress Cataloging-in-Publication Data

Names: Martin, Toby F., editor of compilation. | Weetch, Rosie, editor of compilation.
Title: Dress and society : contributions from archaeology / edited by Toby F. Martin and Rosie Weetch.
Description: Oxford ; Philadelphia : Oxbow Books, 2016. | Includes bibliographical references and index.
Identifiers: LCCN 2016044909 (print) | LCCN 2016045838 (ebook) | ISBN 9781785703157 (paperback) | ISBN 9781785703164 (ePub) | ISBN 9781785703164 (epub) | ISBN 9781785703171 (mobi) | ISBN 9781785703188 (pdf)
Subjects: LCSH: Clothing and dress--Europe--History--To 1500. | Clothing and dress--Social aspects--Europe--History--To 1500. | Identity (Psychology)--Europe--History--To 1500. | Human body--Social aspects--Europe--History--To 1500. | Material culture--Europe--History--To 1500. | Social archaeology--Europe. | Europe--Antiquities.
Classification: LCC GT560 .D74 2016 (print) | LCC GT560 (ebook) | DDC 391.0094--dc23
LC record available at https://lccn.loc.gov/2016044909

All rights reserved. No part of this book may be reproduced or transmitted in any form or by any means, electronic or mechanical including photocopying, recording or by any information storage and retrieval system, without permission from the publisher in writing.

Printed in the United Kingdom by Hobbs the Printers Ltd

For a complete list of Oxbow titles, please contact:

UNITED KINGDOM	UNITED STATES OF AMERICA
Oxbow Books	Oxbow Books
Telephone (01865) 241249, Fax (01865) 794449	Telephone (800) 791-9354, Fax (610) 853-9146
Email: oxbow@oxbowbooks.com	Email: queries@casemateacademic.com
www.oxbowbooks.com	www.casemateacademic.com/oxbow

Oxbow Books is part of the Casemate Group

Front cover: Colour plate from Meyrick, S. R. 1815. The Costume of the Original Inhabitants of the British Islands, from the Earliest Periods to the Sixth Century. London: R. Havell.
Back cover: Umbonate brooch with two rows of 14 cells for enamels found in Hampshire. PAS: HAMP-515B13 (PAS finds reproduced under Creative Commons Share-Alike Agreement).

Contents

List of Figures and Tables v
Preface vii

1. Introduction: dress and society 1
   Toby F. Martin and Rosie Weetch

2. Combination, composition and context: readdressing British Middle Bronze
   Age ornament hoards (*c.* 1400–1100 cal. BC) 14
   Neil Wilkin

3. Personal objects and personal identity in the Iron Age: the case
   of the earliest brooches 48
   Sophia Adams

4. 'Active brooches': theorising brooches of the Roman north-west
   (first to third centuries AD) 69
   Tatiana Ivleva

5. The Roman military belt – a status symbol and object of fashion 94
   Stefanie Hoss

6. Middle Anglo-Saxon dress accessories in life and death: expressions
   of a worldview 114
   Alexandra Knox

7. 'Best' gowns, kerchiefs and pantofles: gifts of apparel in the north-east
   of England in the sixteenth century 130
   Eleanor R. Standley

8. Redressing the balance: dress accessories of the non-elites in Early Modern England 151
Natasha Awais-Dean

9. Cultural presumptions and curatorial context: reassessing the 'highland brooch' of Early Modern Scotland 170
Stuart Campbell

List of Figures and Tables

Figure 2.1. Key examples of British Middle Bronze Age ornaments.
Figure 2.2. The distribution of ornament hoards by metal type.
Figure 2.3. Histogram of the four most common ornament types and sub-types from all hoard deposits.
Figure 2.4. Pie charts of a. ornament types from all hoard deposits and b. 'goldwork only' hoard deposits.
Figure 2.5. The distribution of Sussex Loops in Southern England with detail.
Figure 2.6. a. Object type connections within 'all types' of ornament hoard; b. object type connections within 'gold-work only' ornament hoards; c. object type connections within 'mixed' hoards.
Figure 2.7. The reported spatial relationships between the objects found within the Hollingbury Hoard, Sussex.
Figure 3.1. Parts of an Iron Age bow brooch.
Figure 3.2. Simple typology of Early and Middle Iron Age brooches.
Figure 3.3. Distribution of findspots of Early and Middle Iron Age brooches in Britain.
Figure 3.4. Overview of the context of Early and Middle Iron Age brooches, including excavated and stray finds from known sites.
Figure 3.5. Location and quantity of brooches found in burials.
Figure 4.1. What brooches do in the Roman north-west.
Figure 4.2. A depiction of a woman wearing four brooches found in Neumarkt im Tauchental, Austria.
Figure 4.3. Knee brooch, found in Leeds.
Figure 4.4. Umbonate brooch with two rows of 14 cells for enamels found in Hampshire.
Figure 4.5. Tombstone of a deceased 4-year old Vibius. Found in Hohenstein/Liebenfels, Austria.
Figure 4.6. Tombstone depicting a family with three men wearing disc brooches. Found in Strass in Steiermark, Austria.
Figure 5.1. Funerary monument of the soldier Publius Flavoleius Cordus from Klein-Winternheim (near Mainz/D), dated between 15 and 43 AD.
Figure 5.2. Belt-sets, various dates.
Figure 5.3. Belt-sets, various dates.
Figure 5.4. Funerary monument of an unknown soldier in Istanbul (third century AD), displaying the end of his belt.
Figure 6.1. Location map of sites included in study area of Cambridgeshire and Suffolk. Diamonds indicate documented Minster sites.

Figure 6.2. Distribution of beads and pendants at Bloodmoor Hill, Carlton Colville, Suffolk, in all Saxon phases.
Figure 6.3. Bucket pendants.
Figure 7.1. A youth's decorative dark brown leather jerkin.
Figure 7.2. Remains of the leather pantofle from the Castle Ditch dump at the Black Gate, Newcastle-upon-Tyne.
Figure 7.3. The miniature portrait of Henry Brandon, 2nd Duke of Suffolk, by Hans Holbein the Younger, c. 1541.
Figure 7.4. A linen kerchief.
Figure 8.1. Two views of a gold aglet with ridge and pellet decoration, found in Greenwich, Greater London; England; first half of sixteenth century.
Figure 8.2. Cast and gilded bronze hat ornament depicting Laocoon and his son overcome by a serpent.
Figure 8.3. Gold and enamelled hat ornament set with diamonds, rubies, and possibly a garnet showing the Conversion of Saul; Italy or Spain; mid-sixteenth century.
Figure 8.4. Silver button stamped on the obverse with two hearts surmounted by a crown, found in an unknown parish, Norfolk.
Figure 9.1. Brass brooch from Tomintoul in the eastern highlands of Scotland.
Figure 9.2. Silver and niello brooch from Kengharair on the Isle of Mull.
Figure 9.3. a. Silver and niello brooch from Ballachulish; b. brass example from the eastern highlands of Scotland.
Figure 9.4. Assemblages from burgh and urban sites show that these brooches were used alongside a wide range of mainstream European dress accessories and other items.

Table 2.1. Ornament types in Rowlands' two hoard 'clusters'.
Table 2.2. The numerical relationship between ornaments and tools/weapons in hoards containing both ornaments, tools and/or weapons.
Table 6.1. Sites with dress accessories in either/both the cemetery and settlement areas, and whether the cemetery objects are reflected in the settlement and vice versa.
Table 6.2. Dress accessories at Bloodmoor Hill, comparing settlement finds to grave goods.
Table 6.3. Sites in data set with corresponding cemetery and settlement phasing.
Table 8.1. Comparison of select categories of dress accessories from the post-medieval period between those made of copper-alloy and those declared as Treasure.
Table 8.2. Breakdown of buttons, cufflinks, and dress accessories reported as Treasure from September 1997 to the end of 2009.

Preface

It was surprising to us both when we found out that, having studied for our Masters degrees together, we were both undertaking PhD research into Anglo-Saxon brooches: Toby looking at the cruciform brooches of the early Anglo-Saxon period and Rosie considering the brooches of the later Anglo-Saxon period. As our research progressed we found we were covering similar topics concerning how dress and dress accessories were especially well placed to not only communicate aspects of individual and group identity but also to create that social reality. While we were stimulated by discussions of such matters occurring both within and beyond the field of archaeology, we became frustrated on two levels: first by the lack of communication between researchers of different periods, and second by the lack of archaeological engagement with relevant work happening in other disciplines. We wanted to know how prehistorians thought about dress, how dress historians dealt with material culture, and what archaeology would look like through the lens of Fashion Studies. All groups were dealing with similar source material, albeit from different contexts and time periods, but were the questions we were all asking the same?

In order to satisfy our own curiosity, we held a conference in 2012 called *Rags and Riches: Dress and Dress Accessories in Social Context* with the aim of bringing together archaeologists, historians, and others from related disciplines, regardless of their period of study, to discuss current issues of methodology, theory and interpretation of dress. When the call for papers went out we received over 70 abstracts, a sure sign of the liveliness of the field of dress studies in its broadest sense. Through our very diverse program of speakers, the day-long conference facilitated a multidisciplinary dialogue between researchers studying both historic and contemporary modes of dress. By the end of the day it became clear that we all shared at least two specific areas of current theoretical debate: the ways in which dress can both communicate and create social identities, and dress's unique relationship with the human body. We began using these ideas in our own work, and thought more about how archaeologists could incorporate these ideas into their interpretations of the physical remains of dress that are preserved in the archaeological record. This led to the creation of a session at the *Theoretical Archaeology Group* Conference also in 2012, called *Dressing Sensibly: Sensory Approaches to Dress for Archaeologists*. Inspired by the work of modern fashion theorists who spoke at our original conference, this session focused on the object-body relationships that we felt were less fully explored within archaeology.

All this collaboration and cross-disciplinary discussion had largely considered what other fields could offer archaeologists who studied dress, but this volume has turned the tables to showcase approaches to dress current in archaeology. The volume you have before you now is therefore not an account of the proceedings of either of these events, but this background was fundamental to the topics we decided to include here. We hope that it will spark new ways forward not just for our own field, but also for those who think about dress outside of archaeology.

Toby F. Martin and Rosie Weetch
2016

Chapter 1

Introduction: dress and society

Toby F. Martin and Rosie Weetch

'Fashion is not something that exists in dresses only. Fashion ... has to do with ideas, the way we live, what is happening'. – Coco Chanel

Styles of dress are indeed embedded deeply in society, and as such, they provide ideal subjects for the social archaeologist. Further to the archaeologist's benefit, dress is inescapably material, not just in its rough twills, delicate silks, practical toggles, and ornate jewels, but also in the way its material aspects affect our corporeal experience of the world and its inhabitants through our – more often than not – clothed bodies. In the academic discipline of archaeology, it is chronological and geographical variation of dress styles, technologies and habits that tend to drive our enquiries. They help us to distinguish between this phase and that, or this culture and that one. But the material and social aspects of dress can reveal something of a more meaningful nature than just a useful method of distinguishing and naming archaeological entities. Dress, or perhaps more specifically body ornamentation, is up there with the creation of images at the genesis of what we might recognise as modern human behaviour in the Middle to Upper Palaeolithic transition (White 1992, 539). This chimes with the Biblical account, wherein the first act of humankind was to cover its nudity with fig leaves and animal skins, thereby doubly segregating itself from nature not only by a desire for clothing, but also through the exploitation of the animal and plant worlds to satisfy that need (Genesis 3:6, 3:21). In short, to be human is to be clothed (see Turner [1980] 2012). Indeed, while Jane Goodall's chimps amazed the world in the 1960s with their ability to use simple tools, imagine the reaction had these primates been observed dressed in their own apparel. The notion is absurd, comical even, because it transgresses our preconceptions of what is human and what is animal: dress defines the former, perpetual nudity the latter.

We take a very broad definition of the term 'dress' to include all forms of body ornamentation (for more on definitions see Nicklas and Pollen 2015, 2). Although most of the contributions focus on discrete items such as garments and jewellery, we do not see any fundamental differences, for instance, in the application of certain hairstyles, tattoos or other body modifications often beyond the evidence offered by the archaeological record. 'Dress' does not just refer to the noun that describes the material things we place upon or apply to our bodies, but also the verb that describes the actions, thoughts and motivations behind the shaping of our bodies in the view of both others and ourselves. As such, we might ask what is so special about dress compared with other material culture, and if such a thing as a general archaeological approach to dress exists: does dress perform similar functions and engender similar possibilities in every society?

In this introductory chapter we have chosen to focus upon the subjects of identity and the body, and have asked our contributors to do likewise in their contributions. Beyond the practical functions of garments as a means of survival against the elements, everywhere dress seems to be involved in the creation of similarity and difference, be that based on gender or age, ethnicity, or any other means of distinguishing between some groups whilst uniting others (e.g. Martin 2015). All of these aspects collide under the auspices of identity, a subject that has been of interest to archaeologists for some time now, and is seemingly never far away in archaeological accounts of dress. Dress therefore is about creating both equalities and inequalities between people, and as such, it is often fundamental in the structuring of power relations in society (Peregrine 1991). Furthermore, the specific relationship between identity and dress is inevitably linked with notions of understanding, constructing and experiencing similar or different bodies (Joyce 2005; Turner [1980] 2012). Although the archaeology of dress offers great potential in the dualism between identity and the body, it is by no means limited to this. Rather, these two areas permit archaeologies of dress to communicate with archaeologies of many different kinds of materials, sites or landscapes, and we hope also to academic disciplines beyond our own. For this reason, our introductory chapter begins with an account of the place of dress within the archaeological discipline and beyond it, before moving on to explore what we mean by the involvement of dress in archaeologies of the body and identity.

Dress in archaeology

Given the predominance of items relating to personal adornment in the archaeological record, studies of dress and jewellery have traditionally occupied a surprisingly peripheral position. While the study of textiles tends to be relegated to summary reports or highly specialist volumes and is rarely integrated into broader archaeological discussion, dress accessories, especially metallic ones, are typically favoured by those great compilers of catalogues and corpora: typologists. There are good reasons for this, and the key may lie in the pace at which dress styles tend to progress. While of course this accelerated in the eighteenth and early nineteenth centuries due to new means of industrialised production and fast-moving visual media that could communicate the latest sartorial styles (Flood and Grant 2014), it seems to hold true that in most periods, historic or prehistoric, styles of dress (i.e. fashion) often move faster than other material cultural phenomena, and this may well be due to their inescapable links with human lifespans. The pace of change is a little different for other material culture such as tools, ceramics, buildings, paintings and sculptures and so on which are made to outlive their creators or owners. Hence, links with the body are again tantamount: transitory fashions can perish or adapt alongside ageing and mortal bodies. As such, archaeological dress objects have traditionally made excellent chronological indicators, which helps to explain their popularity in typology, because typology has been, and always will be, used to construct chronologies.

Nevertheless, archaeology has long risked the relegation of dress items to typological and chronological studies, and it is this tendency that this volume was designed to confront and help remedy, with the bold statement that if archaeologists of dress want their work to be more widely relevant and recognised, we must embed our investigations in wider and theoretically informed discussions of society. Because it produces, maintains and sometimes contests the social relations that exist between people, dress is not something that happens *in* society, it *is* society.

Historically speaking, archaeological studies of dress have rarely recognised this fundamental significance of clothing as a means of framing almost every social interaction, with many writers striving more for reconstruction than interpretation. Dress ornaments are extremely prominent among the archaeological remains of virtually every major European period since the Bronze Age. Despite this, there seems to have been a reluctance to include them in mainstream accounts of these societies, not least in terms of how these items were worn, who used them and what the significance of these people and their specific actions may have been. One reason for this this may be that the people who seem to have worn much of the jewellery that tends to survive, at least since the Early Medieval period, were women, and archaeology has historically been inclined to minimise the roles of women and their relationships with material culture in the past (Conkey and Gero 1991; Wylie 1992). There is a general tendency in any case to dismiss anything to do with personal adornment, regardless of the gender of the wearer, as being of the realm of the feminine, perceived as trivial and frivolous, an unfortunate prejudice that stems from present-day attitudes to dress, jewellery and fashion (Taylor 2002, and below). This attitude is exemplified in a quotation from Edward Thurlow Leeds, a renowned early twentieth-century archaeologist best known for his work on the Anglo-Saxon period, who wrote:

> '(e)ven in these early times the subservience of the feminine mind to the dictates of fashion is clearly perceptible, more especially in that most distinctive article of feminine attire – even far back in prehistoric times – the fibula or brooch' (Leeds 1913, 29)

The fact that dress in the past is predominantly studied by female researchers may also have some relevance here (see Gilchrist 1991). Perhaps preoccupations with typology may also be explained as a reaction against the effeminate nature of dress ornaments, typology being a form of hyper-masculinisation, diffusing the effeminate nature of many of these objects in a highly systematised, essentially mathematical structure, effectively banishing the women (more so than men) who actually wore many of these objects into footnotes.

Despite this critique, classificatory studies still produce extremely valuable empirical data, which are of enormous value to the rest of the discipline, and provide perhaps the firmest footings for studies of dress in most periods. Of course, the use to which dress objects are put in archaeological research depends in major part on the available evidence. For instance, the hoard, settlement and mortuary contexts discussed by some of our contributors here, including Wilkin, Adams, Ivleva, Knox and Standley, open up areas of discussion including ritual practice, worldview and gender, among many others. On the other hand, the less than ideal decontextualised dress ornaments in museum collections discussed by Campbell lead to interrogations of the historical and pictorial record, and the same can be said of the metal-detected finds recorded by the Portable Antiquities Scheme discussed by Awais-Dean and Standley. The growth of the Portable Antiquities Scheme has in fact inspired a welcome resurgence in the study of dress items in recent years, with enormous numbers of finds coming to light perhaps from disturbed mortuary and hoard contexts or from casual loss (e.g. Thomas 2000; Awais-Dean 2012; Adams 2013; Kershaw 2013; Standley 2013; Booth 2014; Weetch 2014; Felder 2014; Martin 2015). Again, the decontextualised nature of these metal-detected finds is far from ideal and generally requires analogies to be drawn from the archaeological contexts we do possess, or recourse to literary or pictorial sources (as above). Additionally, these large numbers of finds without context are forcing archaeologists to approach their data in different ways in order to mitigate the kinds of biases this generally poor quality data brings with it (Chester-Kadwell 2009; Robbins 2013).

The papers in this volume showcase the diversity of approaches inspired not only by different types and qualities of data, but also different theoretical and methodological backgrounds. For instance, there are noticeable differences taken between the prehistoric papers by Wilkin and Adams compared to the trio of Early Modern papers by Standley, Awais-Dean and Campbell, with the former emphasising archaeological theoretical approaches, and the latter focusing more upon methodology drawn from the discipline of History. The Roman and Medieval papers by Ivleva, Hoss and Knox display more of a balance between these two ends of the scale. Despite this multiplicity of approaches, the subject matter of dress provides the bridge across the theoretical, methodological and chronological divides. To answer the question posed above concerning whether or not one can delineate a general archaeological approach to dress, we think it is fair to say that such a thing does not exist, and neither would we want to define one, as it would only serve to inhibit communication between researchers of various archaeological periods, already divided by colossal intervals of time. Indeed, we have found the concepts of identity and the body necessary to rein-in the diversity of possibly approaches that archaeologists take to dress. A book like this one is not intended to circumscribe the archaeology of dress, but is intended instead to open this area up to archaeologists with specialist interests elsewhere.

Beyond archaeology

As a discipline that borrows extensively from others, archaeology has contributed surprisingly little to the wider field of dress history. Dress history (after Taylor 2002; 2004) emerged from the discipline of history through the influence of material culture studies, ethnography, fashion studies and social history, and was welcomed especially for bringing attention to social groups historically excluded from traditional histories for reasons to do with social class, gender or ethnicity (Nicklas and Pollen 2015). With strengths in material culture and social history 'from the bottom up', one might have thought archaeology would be in an ideal position to contribute to the general history of dress in the past, but this has not been the case. Dress history is by now a mature discipline, and since the late 1960s the field has had two academic journals: *Costume* (the journal of the Costume Society) and *Textile History*. Despite this long history, a cursory search through the back catalogue of *Costume* reveals only two or three contributions of an explicitly archaeological nature. Indeed, papers concerning any subjects earlier than the seventeenth century are rare. This is perhaps largely due to the fact that the conventional view within dress history is that fashion did not exist before the Renaissance, and that prior to this dress was largely practical and borne out of necessity. The same is broadly true for *Textile History*, though due to its more technical perspective it has a little more to offer in terms of archaeologically recovered textiles. Nevertheless, due to the subject matter of the journal, contributions have tended to focus only on places and periods were textiles are actually preserved, so archaeological contributions naturally focus on Egypt where the climate has been most suitable. Indeed, it seems that the understandable focus on textiles in dress history has acted to perturb archaeologists. As this volume shows, however, textile preservation is by no means a necessity when it comes to talking about dress, and there is therefore little reason for dress history to encroach only rarely on periods earlier than the second millennium AD. Indeed, very few of our papers here rely on evidence from textiles, and tend instead to focus on the metallic remains more favourable to archaeological preservation. Archaeology perhaps stands in a good position to offer up this kind of evidence and means of approaching it to the wider interdisciplinary subject of dress in the past.

Emphasis on materiality as well as on the dress of individuals further down the social scale are already strengths within archaeology, and one can see especially in the contributions here from Standley, Awais-Dean and Campbell that these foci, which stem essentially from the physicality of archaeological remains, complement and confront the written record to interrupt the traditional narratives of dress in the post-medieval period. However, we see little reason why the accounts of Wilkin, Adams, Ivleva, Hoss and Knox should not find their places in an extended dress 'history' of the proto-historic or even prehistoric past. The incidental or highly fragmentary evidence that archaeology offers tends to provoke more quantified or scientific approaches than is generally inspired by pictorial or literary sources. This archaeological methodology, as well as a theoretical focus upon materials and materiality, may well be able to meaningfully contribute to the wider interdisciplinary subject, and we would see such contributions to be, if not entirely novel, at least valuable. Although this is a book written by archaeologists and primarily aimed at archaeologists, we hope that there may be some entry points here for non-archaeologists to explore our discipline, and perhaps borrow from it the slightly different approaches we take.

Bodies and dress in archaeology

Archaeologists have found the field of body-object interactions to be a particularly fertile one (e.g. Meskell 1996; papers in Hamilakis, Pluciennik and Tarlow 2002; Joyce 2005). What better objects to interrogate in this manner than those that ornament, enhance or circumscribe actual bodies? Archaeological research of this nature generally harks back to Marcel Mauss's sociological work on 'techniques of the body' ('*techniques du corps*') published in 1934 (republished and translated in Mauss 1973), in which he established the idea of the human body as a mutable frame that could be taught to move and experience the world in different manners according to its cultural context. The other major touchstone is Judith Butler's *Bodies That Matter* (1993), a philosophical work that had a colossal influence on gender studies, establishing as it did the idea that the male or female body should not be taken for granted as a predetermined default human condition; the anatomical body perceived as male or female was a cultural construction in its own right. The work of both Mauss and Butler is linked by their emphases on the highly variable qualities and meanings of bodies in human thought and practice, and it is this mutability that has opened up the body as a subject of research for many disciplines, not least archaeology.

Wearing particular objects is a means of controlling bodily movements and creating different senses of the world, be they visual, auditory or tactile, as well as screening or displaying aspects of the naked human form according to social conventions (Martin 2014). In fact, dress is fundamental to the creation, maintenance and contestations of those conventions in the first place. A focus on dress therefore emphasises the nature of human interaction as an almost inescapably body-to-body experience (Mathews 2005). Even in a world where virtual communication is beginning to outstrip face-to-face contact, video conferencing is still imbued with a special and unique value. For some time, Turner's idea of dress as a 'social skin' persevered (first published in 1980, reprinted in 2012), suggesting that clothing formed the culturally intelligible façade of the asocial, natural body. For Turner, clothing was symbolic of some inner being, and its function was to display the qualities and meanings of that being to the world. For both Turner and Mauss, the body's morphology, dress and movements were encoded cultural symbols of, among other things, identity (see below). However, the idea of an inner self finds its origins in the Cartesian duality of body and mind as separate entities, with the latter being attributed primacy (Meskell 1996, 3; Thomas 2002). Unsurprisingly therefore, this approach has been met with criticism (see Meskell 1996, 7–8; Gilchrist 2000, 91; Joyce 2005, 151). Archaeologists are probably now more comfortable viewing the formation of meanings associated with dress as performative, or in other words, reliant at least in part with bodily actions. Because of the pre-eminence of corporeality as the site of human experience, bodily adornment cannot be seen as secondary to the construction and display of social meanings, but simultaneous with them (Meskell 2000; Fischer and Loren 2003, 225–6). Dress, therefore, should not be seen as a veil of prefabricated meanings draped passively over the body. Meanings emerge through the repeated and habitual actions of the body; the individual *is* the body. The manners in which people choose to wear garments or ornaments, and how this material culture shapes and gives meaning to bodies, is fundamental and variously explored throughout this volume.

There is of course something very special about objects that are as closely associated with bodies as garments and jewellery. The key to this may well be biography, or the idea that people and things travel along parallel trajectories and, as mentioned above in relation to archaeological chronology, this is especially true for dress items (see Martin 2016). Dress objects, and especially non-perishable metallic ones, have a habit of outliving their wearers, and this creates scenarios in which people have to deal with objects that have become intimately connected with the bodies of their deceased owners, leading to the phenomena of grave goods and heirlooms, to give just two possibilities. Archaeological deposits contain dress objects both still accompanying their wearers in graves as well as apart from them, and the papers in this volume deal with both scenarios. For instance, while Wilkin, Knox and Campbell bear witness to estranged, disembodied dress items found in hoards, settlements and in museum collections, Hoss examines the ways in which the body habits encouraged by large Roman military belts went toward creating masculine, military bodies. Both Standley and Awais-Dean also deal with similarly estranged objects whose ownership is managed and made legitimate through wills and bequests. It is specifically the material affordances of dress items that lead to these complex practices, and this is an area in which archaeology can make substantial contributions. The materiality of dress also leads to quite particular identity formation processes, and it is to this final area that this introductory chapter will now turn.

Identities and dress in archaeology

> 'There is much to support the view that it is clothes that wear us and not we them; we may make them take the mould of arm or breast, but they mould our hearts, our brains, our tongues to their liking.' Virginia Woolf, *Orlando* (1928, 180)

Dress has long been thought to specifically relate to the identity of the wearer. Since the earliest work of culture-historians in the late nineteenth century, the objects people chose to adorn themselves with in the past were considered indicators of ethnicity, age, gender and so on. And while modern archaeologists now view the relationship between objects and identities as far more nuanced than the straightforward passive relationship expounded by these early practitioners (see below), there is a persistent notion that dress, over all other forms of material culture, is especially well placed for the construction and expression of identities (Callmer 2008; Dickinson 1991; Eckardt 2015, 35–50; Effros 2004; Eicher 1995; Harlow 2004, 203; Hides and O'Sullivan 2002; Jundi and Hill 1998; Kershaw 2013; Martin 2015; Parani 2007, 498; Sørensen 1997; Swift 2000; 2004).

The examination and understanding of human identities has been a major research agenda in the social sciences for the last 30 years. In these decades the concept of identity has been redefined. Previous assumptions that genetics and biology were the most significant determinates of what makes a person who they are were challenged. Identity was no longer viewed as a passive set of fixed inherent criteria that people were born with, and instead it was viewed as a fluid cultural construct. It was something that could be chosen, created and manipulated. These new ideas quickly diffused across disciplinary boundaries (Brubaker and Copper 2000, 3) and were particularly influential in archaeology and anthropology in the context of a renewed interest in ethnicity, a topic that had been avoided since the Second World War (Barth 1969; Bently 1987; Shennan 1989; Jones 1997; Graves-Brown et al. 1996). These ideas were exported to other facets of identity, and gender especially saw a revolutionary redefining in light of these arguments (see above).

As archaeologists we are now very familiar with the term identity, but it is a term that is very rarely defined (Brubacker and Copper 2000), indeed it is often assumed that the reader has an instinctive understanding of the word, and it is used in many different ways. Traditionally, archaeologists have tended to use the term identity as a category of analysis, to classify people in the past into various, mutually exclusive, categories including gender, age, belief, and class. In her chapter here, Ivleva questions this uncritical use of the term. There is now a shift in archaeology towards studying identity as a category of practice, as something that is used, created and experienced by individuals in their everyday life. This approach sees identity as a series of situated practices (Meskell 2001, 132–3) in which individual facets (gender, age, class etc.) do not exist in isolation and as such all aspects of identity must be considered simultaneously (Meskell and Preucel 2004, 122).

But unlike social scientists, archaeologists cannot interview their subjects to understand how they practiced identity. They instead have to depend on material remains that survive in the archaeological record (in conjunction with textual sources for those looking at historical periods). Archaeologists studying identity have very often focused on the material remains associated with dress, dress accessories and body ornamentation. The reason we are often drawn to items of dress when exploring past identities is because of the unique relationship between dress and the body (see above), as well as the visual and public nature of dress (Sørensen 1997, 95; Jundi and Hill 1998, 123).

Underpinning the second of these is the idea that dress encodes and expresses information about the identity of the wearer (Lillethun 2011, 189). The idea that dress is communicative and could be therefore be understood as analogous to language became popular in the fields of sociology and psychology in the 1980s (Kaiser 1985; Joseph 1986). These works built on Erving Goffman's idea that social interaction is like a performance and that appearance (including dress) is used by people to convey certain messages about their identity (Goffman [1959] 1990). Also highly influential was Roland Barthes' semiotic 'garment system' in which clothing is understood to encode meaning (Barthes [1964] 1977: 27). By the 1980s and 1990s this chimed with developing archaeological approaches to objects that considered how material culture was like a text to be read and de-coded (Hodder 1986; Shanks and Tilley 1987; Tilley 1990; 1991; Berger 1992; Lele 2006). This semiotic approach remains influential and continues to drive much research into studies of dress (Harlow 2012, 9). But this approach bears a number of limitations, most significantly its tendency to acknowledge the agency of people in their ability to manipulate and create their words, but not the active role of objects in this process (Buchli 2004; Olson 2003, 90; Hicks 2010, 73–4). In this respect Alfred Gell's (1998) posthumously published *Art and Agency: an Anthropological Theory* has been especially influential. Gell argues that objects do not constitute another language and do not have 'meaning', but instead constitute a system of action that changes, rather than encodes, the world (Gell 1998, 6). Material culture, including dress, should be understood as active or as having agency, and therefore it has the ability to construct, maintain, and change social reality, including identities. This concept of object agency has been developed in archaeology and anthropology (Dobres and Robb 2000; Knappett and Malafouris; Dornan 2002; Knappett 2005; Gosden 2005), and is perhaps one of the most influential approaches in terms of the archaeological study of dress and identities. Attention has therefore shifted from considering what dress *means* to what dress *does*, something which all the chapters presented here grapple with.

This links us back to the relationship between the body and dress (see above). Dress is not merely a passive badge that proclaims or encodes the identities of its wearers, it is an embodied practice through which behaviours are learnt and identities are constructed, negotiated and reinforced (Entwistle 2000; Meskell 2000; Butler 1993; Nordbladh and Yates 1990). Identity is more than just something that is represented or expressed, but is something that is experienced through the (clothed) body.

Conclusion

The limitations archaeologists face when dealing with dress in the past are substantial, ranging from the partial survival of different materials in the ground to the selective deposition of different objects by people in the first place. This necessitates that we combine an appreciation of context with an exploitation of theoretical approaches to material culture, identity, and the body, making archaeologists innovative adopters and adaptors of methods and theory borrowed from other academic disciplines, and inventors of some our own. This volume illustrates how objects relating to dress can narrate the stories of individuals and communities alike. Archaeologists explore how dress creates social cohesion and difference, how it influences physical interactions and movement through the world, how it negotiates the creation of social relationships, and, perhaps most fundamentally, how it forms who we are and who we are seen to be. These general points, exemplified by the contributions featured in this book, are testament to the fact that we have moved a long way from the focus on costume reconstruction that characterised traditional work on ancient or historical dress. This earlier work often conflated archaeologies of dress with the romanticised notions of folk dress (i.e. *Tracht*), the noble savage and the pastoral idyll that were cultivated during the nineteenth century, typified perhaps by one of the earliest works on the subject that features on the cover of this book. Reconstruction, however, is no longer a primary goal of dress historians and archaeologists, and neither are typology and chronology. The following chapters show that our focus has since switched to social interpretation, and that archaeological studies of dress have plenty more to offer in this regard.

Bibliography

Adams, S. A. (2013) The First Brooches in Britain: from Manufacture to Deposition in the Early and Middle Iron Age. Unpublished PhD Thesis, University of Leicester.

Awais-Dean, N. (2012) Bejewelled: the Male Body and Adornment in Early Modern England. Unpublished PhD thesis, Queen Mary, University of London.

Barth, F. (1969) *Ethnic Groups and Boundaries: The Social Organization of Culture Difference.* Bergen, Universitetsforlaget; London, Allen & Unwin.

Barthes, R. ([1964] 1977) *Elements of Semiology.* New York, Hill and Wang.

Bentley, G. C. (1987) Ethnicity and practice. *Comparative Studies in Society and History* 29, 24–55.

Berger, A. A. (1992) *Reading Matter: Multidisciplinary Perspectives on Material Culture.* New Brunswick, Transaction Publishers.

Booth, A. L. (2014) Reassessing the Long Chronology of the Penannular Brooch in Britain: Exploring Changing Styles, Use and Meaning Across a Millennium. Unpublished PhD thesis, University of Leicester.

Brubacker, R. and Cooper, F. (2000) Beyond 'identity'. *Theory and Society* 29, 1–47.

Butler, J. (1993) *Bodies That Matter. On the Discursive Limits of "Sex".* London, Routledge.

Buchli, V. (2004) Material culture: current problems. In L. Meskell and R. W. Preucel (eds.) *A Companion to Social Archaeology,* 177–94. Oxford, Blackwell.

Callmer, J. (2008) The meaning of women's ornaments and ornamentation, eastern Middle Sweden in the 8th and early 9th century. *Acta Archaeologia* 79, 185–207.

Chester-Kadwell, M. (2009) *Early Anglo-Saxon Communities in the Landscape of Norfolk.* Oxford, Archaeopress (British Archaeological Reports, British Series, 481).

Conkey, M. W. and Gero, J. M. (1991) Tensions, pluralities and engendering archaeology: an introduction to women and prehistory. In J. M. Gero and M. W. Conkey (eds.) *Engendering Archaeology: Women and Prehistory,* 3–29. Oxford, Blackwell.

Dickinson, T. (1991) Material culture as social expression: the case of Saxon saucer brooches with running spiral decoration. *Studien zur Sachsenforschung* 7, 39–70.

Dobres, M.-A. and Robb, J. E. (2000) *Agency in Archaeology*. London and New York, Routledge.
Dornan, J. (2002) Agency and archaeology: past, present and future directions. *Journal of Archaeological Method and Theory* 9, 303–29.
Eckardt, H. (2015) *Objects and Identities: Roman Britain and the North-Western Provinces*. Oxford, Oxford University Press.
Effros, B. (2004) Dressing conservatively: woman's brooches as markers of ethnic identity? In L. Brubecker and J. Smith (eds.) *Gender in the Early Medieval World: East and West 300-900*, 165–84. Cambridge, Cambridge University Press.
Eicher, J. (1995) Introduction: dress as an expression of ethnic identity. In J. Eicher (ed.) *Dress and Ethnicity*, 1–5. Oxford, Berg.
Entwistle, J. (2000) *The Fashioned Body: Fashion, Dress, and Modern Social Theory*. Cambridge, Polity Press.
Felder, K. (2014) Girdle-Hangers in 5th- and 6th-century England. A Key to Early Anglo-Saxon Identities. Unpublished DPhil thesis, University of Cambridge.
Flood, C. and Grant, S. (2014) *Style and Satire: Fashion in Print 1777-1927*. London, V&A Publishing.
Fisher, G. and Loren, D. D. (2003) Introduction. *Cambridge Archaeological Journal* 13(2), 225–230.
Gell, A. (1998) *Art and Agency: An Anthropological Theory*. Oxford, Clarendon.
Gilchrist, R. (1991) Women's archaeology? Political feminism, gender theory, and historical archaeology. *Antiquity* 65, 495–501.
Gilchrist, R. (2000) Unsexing the body: the interior sexuality of medieval religious women. In R. A. Schmidt and B. L. Voss (eds.) *Archaeologies of Sexuality*, 89–103. London, Routledge.
Goffman, E. ([1959] 1990). *The Presentation of Self in Everyday Life*. London, Penguin.
Gosden, C. (2005) What do objects want? *Journal of Archaeological Method and Theory* 12, 193–211.
Graves-Brown, P., Gamble, C. and Jones, S. (1996) *Cultural Identity and Archaeology: The Construction of European Communities*. London, Routledge.
Hamilakis, Y., Pluciennik, M. and Tarlow, S., eds. (2002) *Thinking Through the Body. Archaeologies of Corporeality*. New York and London, Kluwer/Plenum.
Harlow, M. (2004) Female dress, third-sixth century: the messages in the media? *An Tard* 12, 203–215.
Harlow, M., ed. (2012) *Dress and Identity*. Oxford, Archaeopress (British Archaeological Reports, International Series, 2356).
Hicks, D. (2010) The material-cultural turn: event and effect. In D. Hicks and M. C. Beaudry (eds.) *The Oxford Handbook of Material Culture Studies*, 25–98. Oxford, Oxford University Press.
Hides, S. and O'Sullivan, D. (2002) Dressed to express? Material culture, gender and ethnicity. In M. Donald and L. M. Hurcombe (eds.) *Gender and Material Culture in Historical Perspective*, 76–96. Basingstoke, Macmillan.
Hodder, I. (1986) *Reading the Past: Current Approaches to Interpretation in Archaeology*. Cambridge, Cambridge University Press.
Jones, S. (1997) *The Archaeology of Ethnicity: Constructing Identities in the Past and Present*. London, Routledge.
Joseph, N. (1986). *Uniforms and Nonuniforms: Communication through Clothing* New York, Greenwood.
Joyce, R. A. (2005) Archaeology of the body. *Annual Review of Anthropology* 34, 139–58.
Jundi, S. and Hill, J. D. (1998) Brooches and identities in first century AD Britain: more than meets the eye? In C. Forcey J. Hawthorne and R. Witcher (eds.) *TRAC 97: Proceedings of the Seventh Annual Theoretical Roman Archaeology Conference Nottingham 1997*, 125–37. Oxford, Oxbow Books.
Kaiser, S. B. (1985) *The Social Psychology of Clothing and Personal Adornment*. New York, Macmillan.
Kershaw, J. (2013) *Viking Identities: Scandinavian Jewellery in England*. Oxford, Oxford University Press.
Knappett, C. (2005) *Thinking through Material Culture: An Interdisciplinary Perspective*. Philadelphia, University of Pennsylvania Press.
Knappett, C. and Malafouris, L., eds. (2008) *Material Agency: Towards a Non-Anthropocentric Approach*. New York, Springer.
Leeds, E. T. (1913) *The Archaeology of the Anglo-Saxon Settlements*. Oxford, Clarendon Press.

Lele, V. P. (2006) Material habits, identity, semiotic. *Journal of Social Archaeology* 6, 48–70.

Lillethun, A. (2011) Fashion and identity: introduction. In L. Welters and A. Lillethun (eds.) *The Fashion Reader: Second Edition*, 189–92. Oxford and New York, Berg.

Martin, T. F. (2014) (Ad)Dressing the Anglo-Saxon body: corporeal meanings and artefacts in early England. In P. Blinkhorn and C. Cumberpatch (eds.) *The Chiming of Crack'd Bells: Recent Approaches to the Study of Artefacts in Archaeology*, 27–38. Oxford, Archaeopress (British Archaeological Reports, International Series, 2677).

Martin, T. F. (2015) *The Cruciform Brooch and Anglo-Saxon England*. Woodbridge, Boydell and Brewer.

Martin, T. F. (2016) The lives and deaths of people and things: biographical approaches to dress in early Anglo-Saxon England. In R. F. W. Smith and G. L. Watson (eds.) *Writing the Lives of People and Things, AD 500-1700*, 67–87. Farnham, Ashgate.

Matthews, S. (2005) The materiality of gesture: intimacy, emotion and technique in the archaeological study of bodily communication. Open Semiotics Research Centre. Available at: http://www.semioticon.com/virtuals/archaeology/materiality.pdf [accessed March 2016].

Mauss, M. ([1934] 1973) Techniques of the body. *Economy and Society* 2, 70–88.

Meskell, L. (1996) The somatization of archaeology: institutions, discourses, corporeality. *Norwegian Archaeological Review* 29(1), 1–16.

Meskell, L. (2000) Writing the body in archaeology. In A. E. Rautman (ed.) *Reading the Body: Representations and Remains in the Archaeological Record*, 13–21. Philadelphia, University of Pennsylvania Press.

Meskell, L. (2001) Archaeologies of identity. In I. Hodder (ed.) *Archaeological Theory Today*, 187–231. Cambridge, Polity Press.

Meskell, L. and Preucel, R. W. (2004) Identities. In L. Meskell and R. W. Preucel, R. W. (eds.) *A Companion to Social Archaeology*, 121–41. Oxford, Blackwell.

Nicklas, C. and Pollen, A. (2015) Introduction: dress history now: terms, themes and tools. In C. Nicklas and A. Pollen (eds.) *Dress History: New Directions in Theory and Practice*, 1–14. London, Bloomsbury.

Nordbladh, J. and Yates, T. (1990) This perfect body, this virgin text. In I. Bapty and T. Yates (eds.) *Archaeology after Structuralism: Post-Structuralism and the Practice of Archaeology*, 223–37. London, Routledge.

Olsen, B. (2003) Material culture after text: re-membering things. *Norwegian Archaeological Review* 36, 87–104.

Parani, M. (2007) Defining personal space: dress accessories in Late Antiquity. In L. Levan, E. Swift and T. Putzeys (eds.) *Objects in Context, Objects in Use: Material Spatiality in Late Antiquity*, 497–525. Leiden and Boston, Brill.

Peregrine, P. (1991) Some political aspects of craft production. *World Archaeology* 23(1), 1–11.

Robbins, K. (2013) Balancing the scales: exploring the variable effects of collection bias on data collected by the Portable Antiquities Scheme. *Landscapes* 14(1), 54–72.

Shanks, M. and Tilley, C. Y. (1987) *Social Theory and Archaeology*. Cambridge, Polity.

Shennan, S. J., ed. (1989). *Archaeological Approaches to Cultural Identity*, London and New York, Routledge.

Standley, E. R. (2013) *Trinkets and Charms: The Use, Meaning and Significance of Dress Accessories 1300–1700*. Oxford, Oxford University School of Archaeology (Oxford University of Oxford School of Archaeology Monograph 78).

Sørensen, M. L. (1997) Reading dress: the construction of social categories and identities in Bronze Age Europe. *Journal of European Archaeology* 5, 93–114.

Swift, E. (2000) *Regionality in Dress Accessories in the Late Roman West*. Montagnac, M. Mergoil.

Swift, E. (2004) Dress accessories, culture and identity in the Late Roman Period. *An Tard* 12, 217–22.

Taylor, L. (2002) *The Study of Dress History*. Manchester, Manchester University Press.

Taylor, L. (2004) *Establishing Dress History*. Manchester, Manchester University Press.

Thomas, G. (2000) A Survey of Late Anglo-Saxon and Viking-Age Strap-Ends from Britain. Unpublished PhD thesis, University College London.

Thomas, J. (2002) Archaeology's humanism and the materiality of the body. In Y. Hamilakis, M. Pluciennik, and S. Tarlow (eds.) *Thinking Through the Body. Archaeologies of Corporeality*, 29–45. New York and London, Kluwer/Plenum.

Tilley, C. (1990) *Reading Material Culture: Structuralism, Hermeneutics and Post-Structuralism*. Oxford, Basil Blackwell.

Tilley, C. Y. (1991) *Material Culture and Text: The Art of Ambiguity*. London and New York, Routledge.

Turner, T. S. ([1980] 2012) The social skin. *Hau: Journal of Ethnographic Theory* 2(2), 486–504.

Weetch, R. (2014) Brooches in Late Anglo-Saxon England within a North West European Context. A Study of Social Identities between the Eighth and Eleventh Centuries. Unpublished PhD thesis, Reading University.

White, R. (1992) Beyond art: toward an understanding of the origins of material representation in Europe. *Annual Review of Anthropology* 21, 537–64.

Wylie, A. (1992) The interplay of evidential constraints and political interests: recent archaeological research on gender. *American Antiquity* 57(1), 15–35.

Chapter 2

Combination, composition and context: readdressing British Middle Bronze Age ornament hoards (c. 1400–1100 cal. BC)

Neil Wilkin

Introduction

A new range of copper-alloy and gold dress accessories are found in a large number of burials and hoards across North-west Europe during the Middle Bronze Age. By comparison with the fashions of Chalcolithic and Early Bronze Age periods, the ornaments of the Middle Bronze Age are greater in weight but not in surface area and are more plentiful but also more standardised (*cf.* Sørensen 1997, 101; 2013, 229). The socio-cultural context of this change requires attention: the new ornaments allowed individuals and groups to distinguish their identities on gender, status and regional lines, with important overlaps in terms of similarity and difference between individuals and regions (*cf.* Wels-Weyrauch 1989; Sørensen 2013, 230). In central Europe and Scandinavia, ornaments are recorded on the body in funerary contexts (Bergerbrant 2007; Bergerbrant *et al.* 2013; Harris 2012; Randsborg and Christensen 2006), whereas the British evidence is overwhelmingly dominated by hoard deposits belonging to the period known as the 'Ornament Horizon' (c. 1400–1100 BC; 'ornament hoard' hereafter; Fig. 2.1).

This paper develops the understanding of Middle Bronze Age ornament hoards in new directions based on a revised and critically reviewed dataset of hoard deposits (Appendix 2.1). It follows Rowlands (1976) in placing greater emphasis on the composition of hoards, the conceptual relationships between object 'types', and on their spatial relationships, which may reveal patterning and rationale behind acts of deposition (*cf.* Richards and Thomas 1984; Garrow and Gosden 2012, 155–93). It also addresses the evidence for intentional destruction and theories that seek to account for why fragmentation occurred in the course of ritualised metalwork deposition (*cf.* Chapman 2000; Dietrich 2014; Dietrich and Mörtz forthcoming). These approaches inform a discussion of how conceptions of the body and identity changed during

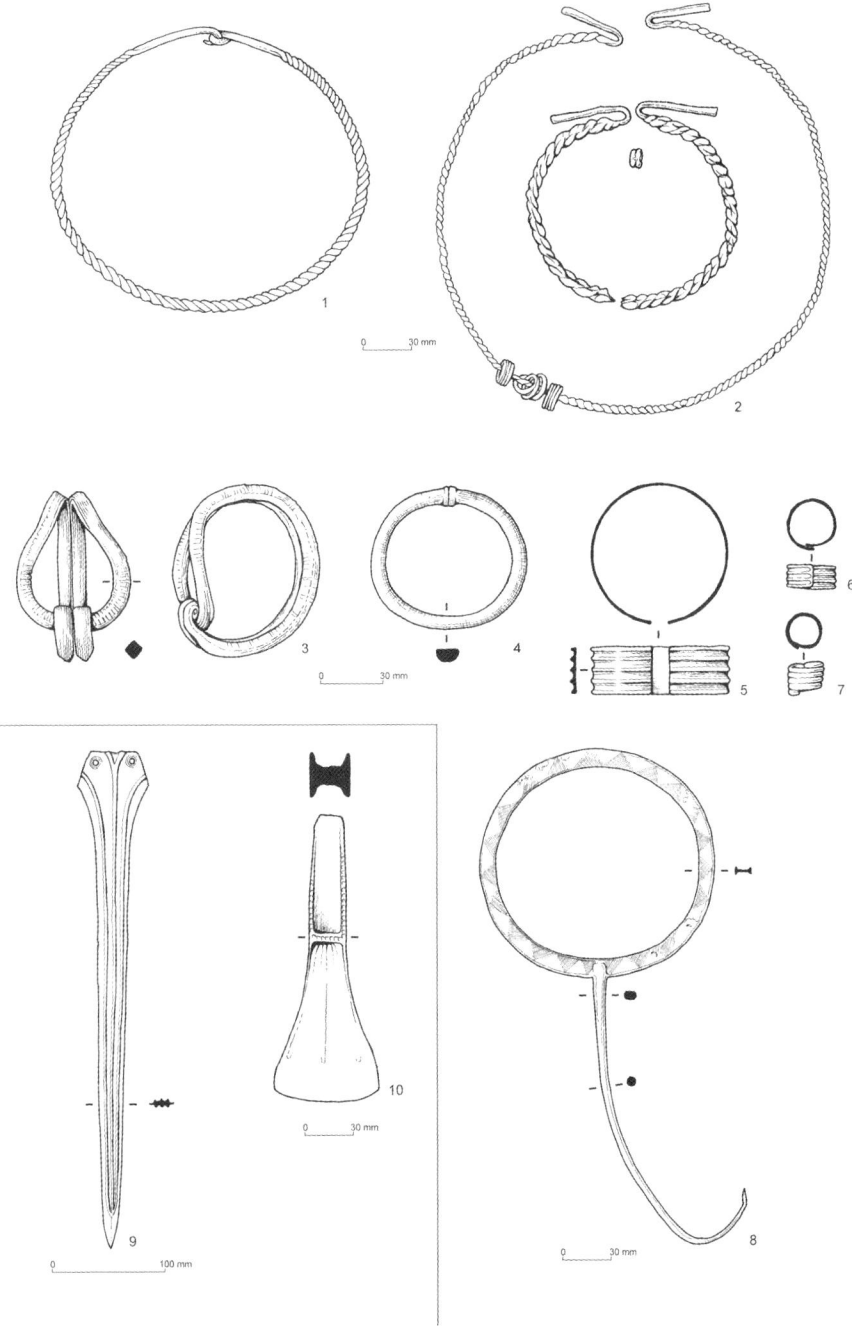

Fig. 2.1: Key examples of British Middle Bronze Age ornaments (drawn by Craig Williams). 1. Spiral twisted torc; 2. Flanged and bar torcs (with threaded rings); 3. Sussex Loop; 4. Bracelet/armring (annular); 5. Cast, ribbed bracelet; 6. Finger-ring (cast, ribbed); 7. Finger-ring (spiral); 8. Pin (quoit headed); 9. Weapon (dirk/rapier); 10. Tool (palstave).

the Bronze Age, with particular reference to the role of hoard deposition during the final centuries of the second millennium cal. BC. It is now commonly accepted that Bronze Age hoards are not the accidentally accrued debris of everyday life but rather a considerable proportion, if not all, are meaningful, structured deposits created in the course of ritualised practices (*cf.* Fontijn 2002; Bradley 2013; Dietrich 2014). The results of this study support that general conclusion but also warn against overly simplistic, one size fits all explanations of hoarding practices. Rather, ornament hoards are best understood with reference to the social and ritual importance of dress in their chronological and geographical context.

Middle Bronze Age ornament hoards: definitions, distribution and chronology

British ornament hoards can be dated typologically to the Taunton and Penard metalwork assemblages (*c.* 1400–1150 cal. BC) which are part of the Middle Bronze Age in conventional terminology (*c.* 1500–1100 cal. BC) (Burgess 1980; O'Connor 1989; Needham 1996; Rohl and Needham 1998; *cf.* Roberts *et al.* 2013, 22–5). The Taunton hoards are composed mainly of bronze objects and concentrated in southern England, while Penard ornament hoards are predominantly gold and more widespread (Roberts 2007) (Fig. 2.2). Smith (1959a) interpreted the deposition of hoards composed of relatively similar ornaments (without parallel among the metal assemblages of preceding centuries) as evidence for a relatively rapid and continentally-inspired 'Ornament Horizon'. The usefulness of the term as a catch-all for ornaments of this date has now been questioned. Both Needham (1990, 263) and Roberts (2007, 148) have argued that refinements in the dating of particular hoards is possible with respect to typology and material, principally the prominence of gold ornaments in later, Penard period, hoards. A cautious distinction is therefore made in the analysis that follows between hoards of the Taunton (*c.* 1400–1250 cal. BC) and Penard (*c.* 1300/1250–1150/1100 cal. BC) phases. These phases do, however, appear to have overlapped and their relationship is currently based on patterns of association rather than absolute dating evidence (B. Roberts pers. comm.). The relationship between these groups or phases receives considerable attention in the analysis and discussion that follows.

Hoards are defined here as two or more closely associated objects from single deposits, even if only one of the objects was an ornament (e.g. a torc associated with a tool). More complex deposits that do not fulfil these criteria are also noted below, the recognition of these (e.g. multiple but apparently related single deposits in close proximity) is set to increase as more discoveries are made through archaeological fieldwork. Hoards have been prioritised over single finds as they provide context and opportunity to identify meaningful relationships and patterning that Garrow and Gosden have recently described as 'networks in which ... items of material culture came to be caught up' (2012, 156). A distinction is also drawn between 'less certain' and 'more certain' hoard deposits (Appendix 2.1). The former are groups of objects

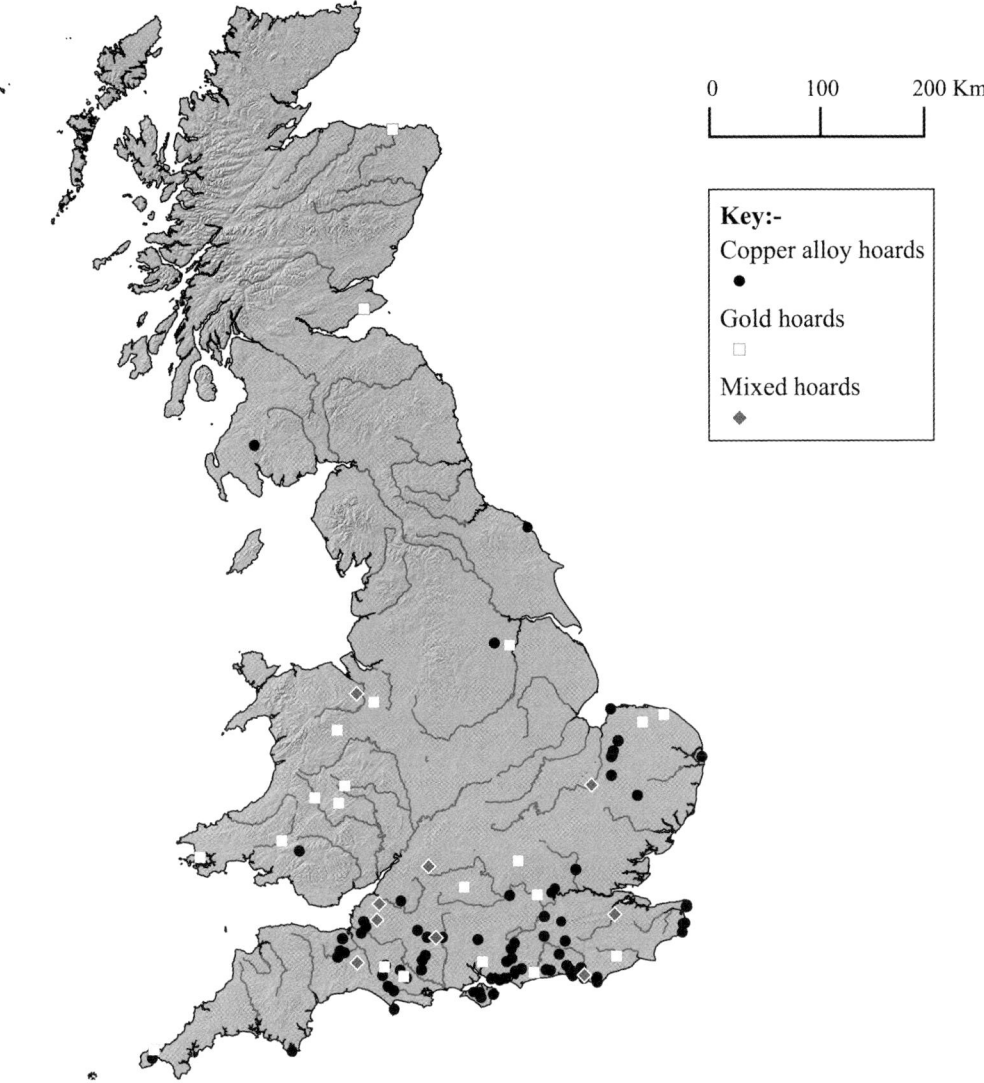

Fig. 2.2: The distribution of ornament hoards by metal type.

that have come down to us as closed hoards but for which no published reference to the group having been found in a single, closed deposit exists or that were found as dispersed hoards in the course of metal detecting. The distinction is not laboured but does, on several occasions, provide a useful way of minimising the danger of biases deriving from problematic recording and recovery. Single finds are not discussed in detail in this paper, although they are of considerable importance and may have been intentionally deposited as well as accidentally lost. A future study designed to integrate ornament hoards and single finds is anticipated.

Two points are important when considering the changing significance of Bronze Age dress and appearance through time. Firstly, the transition from inhumation to cremation as the burial mode of choice, the latter increasingly popular after c. 2100/2000 cal. BC, and dominant by c. 1800/1700 cal. BC (cf. Needham 2005; Sheridan 2007; Needham et al. 2010). This situation is at variance with the continental European evidence where inhumation burial remains popular in many regions and ornaments are found adorning the bodies of the dead during the equivalent Middle Bronze Age, not shifting to cremation burial until the Later Bronze Age (Sørensen 2013, 230–1). The second key point is the shift in the dominant source of archaeological evidence from burial contexts (from c. 2500–1500 cal. BC) to hoard deposits and single finds of metalwork (from c. 1500/1400–700 cal. BC). Only a relatively small number of Middle Bronze Age burials contained ornaments as grave goods, with only four meeting the criteria of 'hoard' defined above (Appendix 2.1, nos. 35, 37, 71 and 98).

Hoard size and biases of preservation and recovery

Most ornament hoards (c. 65%) are relatively small, containing six or fewer objects. Counting only the ornaments from these hoards produces a similar pattern: 74% of all hoards and 69% of 'more certain' hoards contain six or fewer objects. The largest hoards tend to consist of objects made of copper alloy only or of a mixture of copper alloy and gold rather than being exclusively composed of gold ornaments. Of the six hoards containing more than 18 objects, five have been discovered since the introduction of the Treasure Act (1996), which suggests that they are under-represented. The recent discovery of the Wylye Hoard, Wiltshire, apparently deposited in two separate pits (Treasure report 2012 T786), demonstrates how metal detectors can more easily identify large, albeit still relatively rare, ornament hoards.[1]

The evidence of clothed bodies from the funerary contexts of Central Europe suggests that multiple ornaments could be worn together as elaborate costumes (e.g. Wels-Weyrauch 1989). This does not apply equally to all ornament types. It is more likely that an individual wore multiple bracelet/arm-rings than multiple torcs (cf. ibid.). In the case of spiral twisted torcs from ornament hoards in Britain, just over 50% were deposited in groups of two or more. Thus ornament hoards, while generally relatively small, cannot *all* be taken as the costumes of single individuals whose remains are buried elsewhere. Rather they have their own character and significance that needs to be accounted for on its own terms.

Copper-alloy, gold and 'mixed' hoards

Among the 102 ornament hoards considered in this study, 68% consisted of copper-alloy objects only, 23% of gold objects only and 9% were mixed hoards, comprising of objects of copper alloy and gold. Important differences in the distribution of gold and copper-alloy hoards are further discussed below, and it can also be noted that the mixed hoards form a relatively homogeneous group, comprising primarily ornaments of gold associated with a tool or weapon of copper alloy. Thus, as Roberts (2007, 147) has noted, gold and copper-alloy ornaments were rarely mixed within hoards, suggesting the existence of a chronological and/or symbolic difference in how they were perceived. The only recorded exception is the Near Lewes hoard, Sussex (Appendix 2.1, no. 82; Treasure report 2011 T192), which includes four rare gold discs, and may 'prove the rule', as it was deposited in a region where other idiosyncratic decisions were taken, most notably the development of the regionally-specific bracelet type known as the Sussex Loop.

Ornament types

Rowlands (1976, 84–98) distinguished four main categories of ornament: pins, torcs, bracelets/arm-rings and finger-rings, but noted that these masked considerable variation (Fig. 2.3; Appendix 2.2). To this set of divisions, a fifth, 'miscellaneous other', category has been added for the following analysis.

Bracelets/arm-rings and torcs are the most common ornament types from hoard deposits (60% and 45% of hoards, respectively), with pins and finger-rings less well represented (21% and 15% of hoards, respectively, Figs. 2.3 and 2.4). The picture for copper-alloy and gold hoards is similar, but in the case of goldwork only hoards pins are not represented and torcs (especially flange-twisted types) are much more common (Fig. 2.3). The following sections investigate patterns within and between these key types.

Bracelets/arm-rings

Among the bracelets/arm-rings from hoards, annular and penannular forms without further twisting or modifications of form are common (48 of 82: 59%). This pattern is even clearer in the case of goldwork only hoards (Appendix 2.2). A small but significant number of bracelets/arm-rings are more elaborate: spiral twisting (of the same technique as torcs) is a feature of nine of the hoards. The elaborate working of bars into Sussex Loops is a feature of another ten hoards. These armlets are a clear example of the regional expression of identity, occurring within a limited geographical region (Fig. 2.5).

Twenty bracelets/arm-rings of annular and penannular form are decorated with incised designs and a number of Sussex Loops were also marked with repeated vertical nicks, a type of decoration also found on finger-rings and pins. Ribbed bracelets are also among the most accomplished metalwork finds from hoards of this period and in several instances form sets with finger-rings in terms of both form and decoration.

Torcs

There is a clear distinction between the techniques and materials used to make the ornaments grouped here as 'torcs'. Flange twisted torcs with prominent recurved

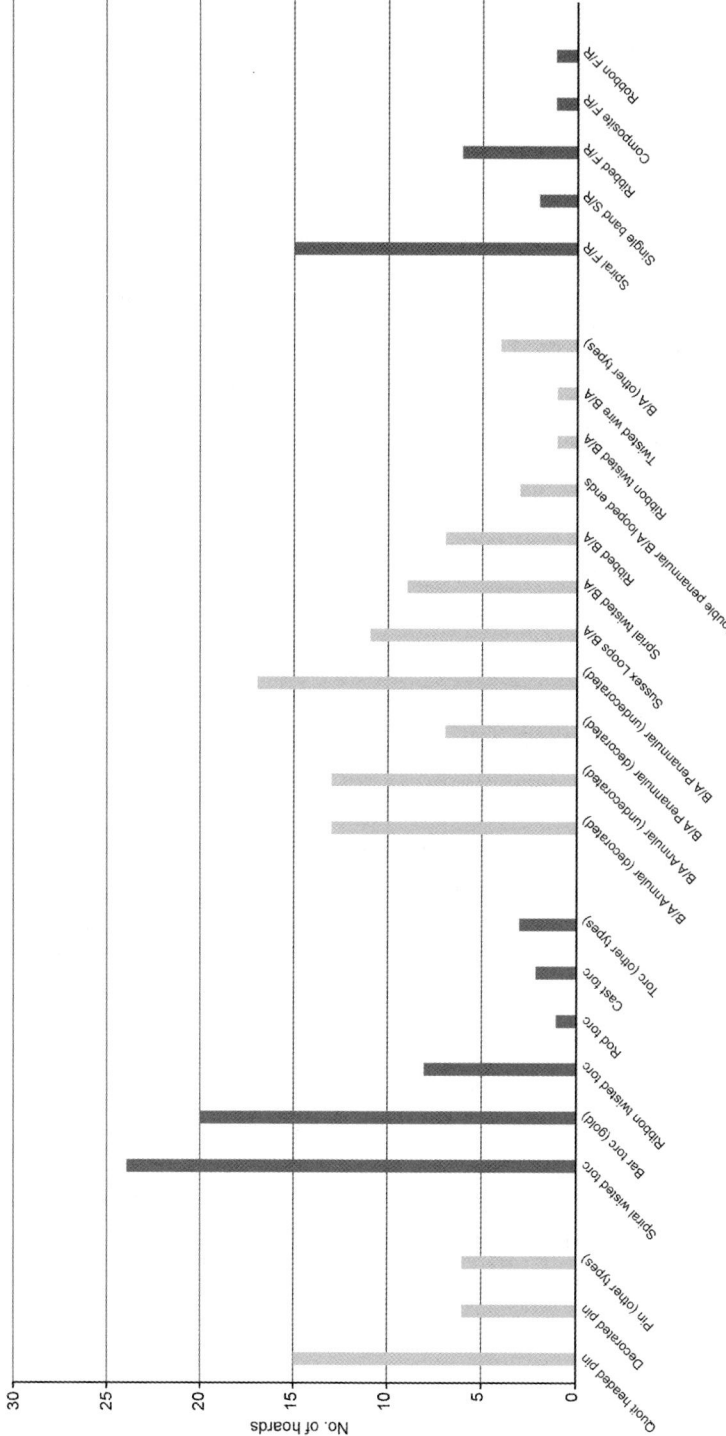

Fig. 2.3: Histogram of the four most common ornament types and sub-types from all hoard deposits (Key:- B/A: Bracelet/armring; F/R: finger-ring).

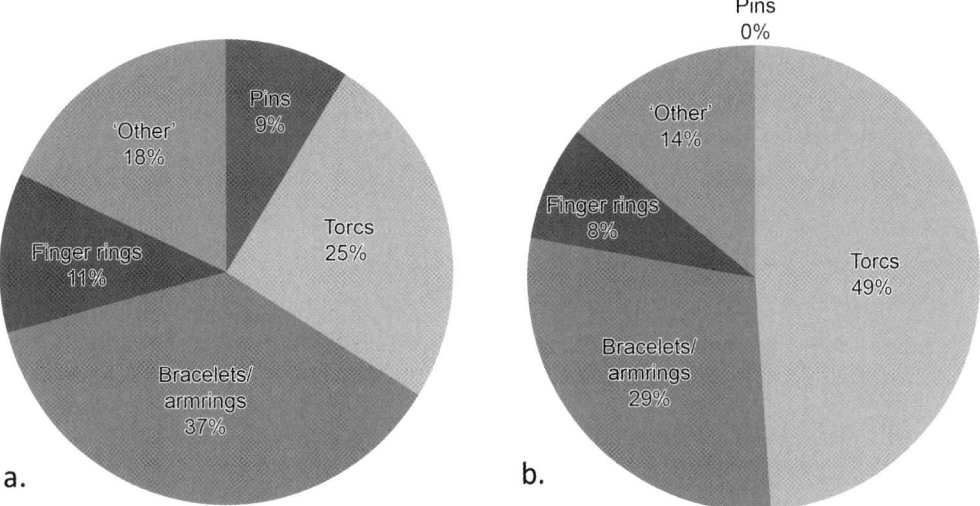

Fig. 2.4: Pie charts of a. ornament types from all hoard deposits and b. 'goldwork only' hoard deposits (see Appendix 2.2 for details).

terminals (also known as 'bar' or 'Tara' torcs: Eogan 1967) appear to have been made exclusively of gold (19 examples), and are generally found with other gold objects (Appendix 2.2). In contrast, spiral-twisted torcs are of copper alloy and are generally found in hoards with other objects of the same material. The technique used to make different torc types differs, as does their length. Some flange-twisted torcs are long enough (and deposited in a coiled fashion) to suggest they were wrapped around an arm, a leg or that they served as girdles around the waist (*ibid.*, 132). The malleability of gold appears to have enabled these different properties to be realised. By contrast, copper-alloy torsion-twisted torcs were worn exclusively around the neck. As noted above, the distinction between gold and copper alloy has been recognised as a spatial and typo-chronological feature and in the size of hoards, but it also had implications for how objects were used.

Untwisted torcs are rare, although it is still to be demonstrated by detailed examination that all twisted torcs were indeed created by means of torsion twisting. There are only two examples of copper-alloy torcs from hoard deposits that were certainly not made by twisting bars of copper alloy or gold. This is notable given that bracelets/arm-rings often found in direct association with torcs were simpler, untwisted forms. This suggests that metalwork made to be worn on different parts of the body had to be made in particular ways, with little room for experimentation or diversion from normative patterns of production.

Pins

Among pins, the most popular type from hoard deposits is the quoit-headed pin, some of which are exceptionally long with very large circular and oval heads which may have

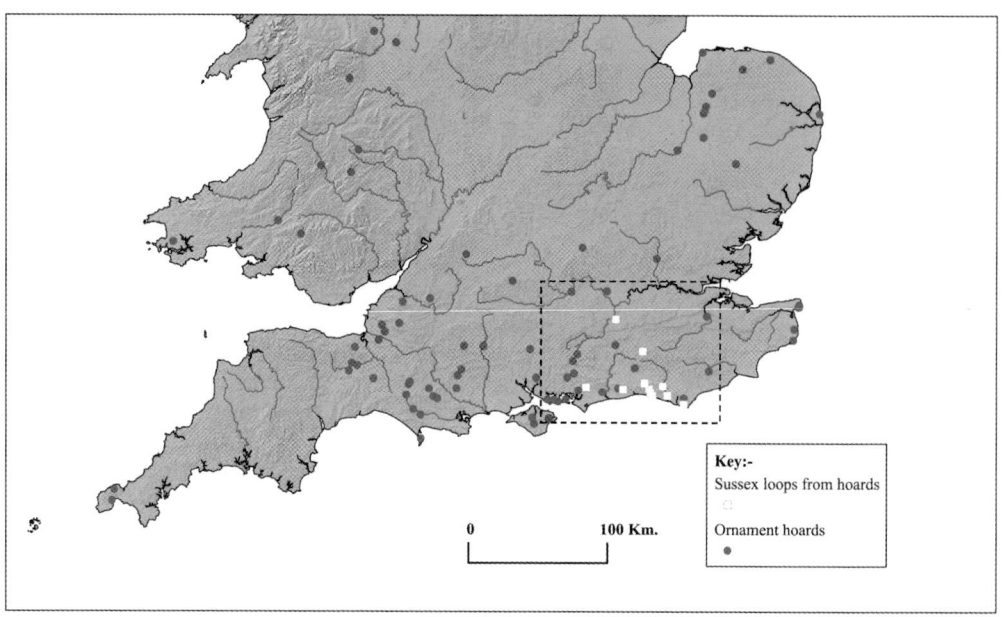

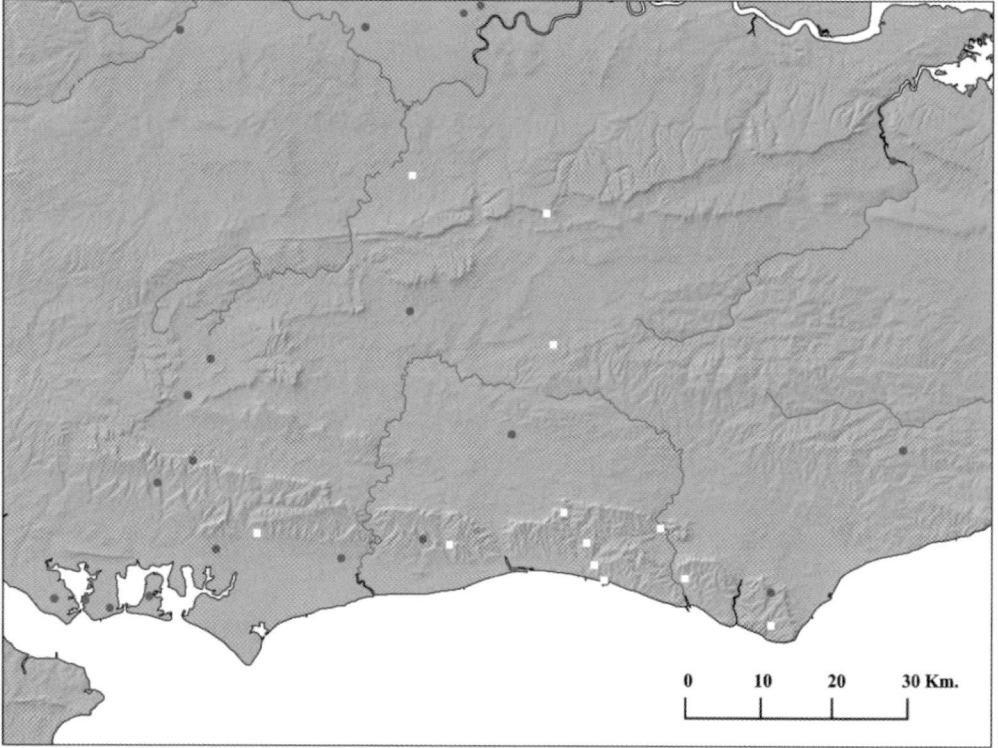

Fig. 2.5: The distribution of Sussex Loops in Southern England, with detail.

served to hold and secure garments such as cloaks (Lawson 1979). A number of these pins carry decoration, as do the decorated (or 'Picardy') pins, although the decorative designs differ between the two types. In two cases, both from very close-by in Norfolk, at Barton Bendish and Boughton Fen, the decoration of quoit-headed pins consists of incised chevrons. The composition of the two hoards is also similar: the Barton Bendish hoard contained two palstaves and knife, while the Boughton Fen hoard (although of the 'less certain' category) is said to have contained two spearheads (Lawson 1979). They therefore appear to represent a localised fashion. Their decoration is unique to the quoit-headed type but in most other cases the decoration of repeated vertical nicks it is also found on bracelet/arm-rings and finger-rings (Rowlands 1976, 87).

Pins are exceptional among the ornament types as they could be worn through or on clothing and cloth, while the majority of the other types were worn directly on or against the body. Indeed, there are only nine examples of decorative fittings that could be mounted or sewn to clothing or other objects. This places the majority of ornaments under study at a remove from perishable clothing and may thus have given pins different connotations compared to the vast majority of ornament types. A higher proportion of pins have been found as single finds than any of the other main object types under study (21 hoards, 45 as single finds compared to bracelets/armlets: 61 hoards, 33 from single finds), perhaps reflecting patterns of casual loss, but also, potentially, different depositional practices.

Finger-rings
The principal finger-ring types are copper-alloy spiral types, worked into coils that overlap two or three times and sometimes from twisted lengths of bar (possibly re-worked torcs or bracelets/arm-rings). Several spiral rings carry decoration of 'nicks' similar to bracelets and armlets. They were thus decorated using similar techniques to Sussex Loops and annular and penanaular bracelets/arm-rings. The rings from the Edington Burtle (Smith 1959b, GB. 44 2(1) and 2(2)) and the Wylye hoards (Treasure report 2012 T786), both from Wiltshire, are miniature versions of ribbed bracelets from the same hoards. On several occasions rings were found looped over torcs prior to being deposited, a practice that is discussed in greater detail below.

Discussion
From this brief overview of the key ornament types, links between types (or sets) have been observed, particularly between finger-rings and bracelets/arm-rings. Different types of ornament, designed for different parts of the body, were made using different techniques and were governed by relatively strict prescriptions regarding how they should appear and whether/how to decorate them. Finally, it was observed that most ornaments were worn against the exposed areas of the body (the neck, arms and fingers), with only pins securing clothing. The extreme size of most quoit-headed pins is therefore of note, suggesting that clothing was elaborated with metalwork only exceptionally, perhaps only in the coldest parts of the day or year. A higher

proportion of pins were deposited as single finds than in hoards and this may reflect different attitudes to depositional practices.

Tool and weapon types

Ornament hoards in fact contain a considerable number of objects best described as tools (41 hoards) and weapons (16 hoards), with a small number containing both (eight hoards: 8%). Palstaves are the most common tool type (30 hoards) from hoards, with most (70%) containing more than one. It is likely that some tools and weapons were worn or carried as dress accessories and personal ornaments. The decorated rapier hilt plate from the Blackrock hoard, Sussex, is a case in point (Piggott 1949; Burgess and Gerloff 1981, pl. 131A). Such objects are, however, in the minority, and relatively plain tools are much more common and there are few instances of the male warrior aesthetic and identity found in some regions of Continental Europe during the Bronze Age (*cf.* Traherne 1995). This, however, does not mean that the tools and weapons included did not have their own symbolic significance. The key point is that they referenced or cited a range of behaviours and tasks that differentiated them from ornaments (*cf.* Fontijn 2002, 239). It was noted above that in Continental Europe ornaments are usually associated with female burials. Palstaves could represent male activity and identity but the case is not clear cut. The possibility of gendered distinctions and combinations within ornament hoards is further discussed below.

The combination of object types

Garrow and Gosden (2012, 167–9) have recently demonstrated the value of highlighting connections between different object types within Iron Age hoards, in addition to quantifying the prevalence of particular types of object. The data presented in Figure 2.5 follows this approach in order to visually present the association between the principal object types (as defined above) from all types of Middle Bronze Age hoard. The 'miscellaneous other' category of ornament has not been included in this analysis as it is not a coherent object type in its own right, although it is included in the analysis when considering whether single object types were deposited alone. In most cases object types are combined within ornament hoards, with most of these containing two or three object types. The regular occurrence of combinations of object types is, in itself, of note and suggests that ornaments selected for deposition were generally not sorted into particular types before deposition, unlike contemporary palstave only hoards (Rowlands 1976, 99–114).

The key object type relationships are between bracelets/arm-rings and tools; bracelets/arm-rings and torcs; and torcs and tools (Fig. 2.6). There are a number of relationships that are notable due to their rarity, principally between finger-rings and pins and between finger-rings and weapons. The former is a feature of only four hoards West Ashling, Sussex (British Museum archive; B. O'Connor pers. comm.);

Barton Bendish, Norfolk (Smith 1959b, GB 7,2 (1–2); Wylye, Wiltshire, Treasure report 2012 T786); Near Lewes, Sussex (Treasure report 2011 T192). All four hoards contained quoit-headed pins and all four are among the five hoards that contain (the same) five object types. It is possible that there was an inability, due to chronological factors, or reluctance due to social/ritual factors, to directly associate finger-rings and pins. In the case of the Wylye hoard, Wiltshire, the pin and finger-rings were found in separate deposits a few metres apart, while the lozenge-headed and quoit-headed pins from both the near Sussex hoard and West Ashling were deposited in a fragmentary state. Only the Barton Bendish hoard contained an intact pin, but relatively little is known about the details of its deposition.

The most common object types deposited on their own are bracelets/arm-rings and torcs, with very few instances of finger-rings and pins deposited alone (Fig. 2.6). Although this is largely consistent with the relative quantity of object types from ornament hoards, goldwork only hoards account for a considerable proportion of the torc only hoards (7 of 12, Fig. 2.6).

Among the goldwork only hoards, the key relationship is clearly between bracelets/arm-rings (mostly penannular/annular bracelets) and torcs (mostly the flange-twisted sub-type). The goldwork only hoards therefore form a relatively coherent and well-defined group (Fig. 2.6). The connections between objects within mixed hoards is similar because, as noted above, almost all of the ornaments within mixed hoards are of gold, while only the tool (often a palstave) is of copper alloy (Fig. 2.6). Thus the evidence for artefact combinations further contributes to Robert's (2007, 148) argument for a distinction between copper-alloy and gold ornament hoards, which may have had significance in terms of chronology or cultural and symbolic differences (e.g. relating to differences in the colour of the metal).

The composition of ornament hoards

There is considerable variety in the combination of object types within ornament hoards: the particular composition of a large number of hoards (*c.* 48%) occurs only once or twice. The remaining hoards belong to only eight composition variants, only one of which contains more than two object types. Variation and complexity is particularly apparent in the case of 'copper-alloy only' hoards and appears to reflect greater flexibility in the rules governing the composition of these hoards compared to 'gold only' hoards (Appendix 2.2).

Rowlands (1976, 11) proposed that the contents of copper-alloy hoards could be arranged into two principal clusters: a complex of hoards containing a range of ornaments with spiral-twisted forms (principally spiral-twisted torcs; 'ST hoards', hereafter) and a second complex with a particular focus on bracelets/arm-rings (*ibid.*; 'other' hoards', hereafter). In the latter case, Rowlands identified three sub-groups, most notably the group of Sussex Loop hoards, and it therefore represents a less well-defined group than the spiral-twisted hoards. Rowlands (*ibid.*) also noted a

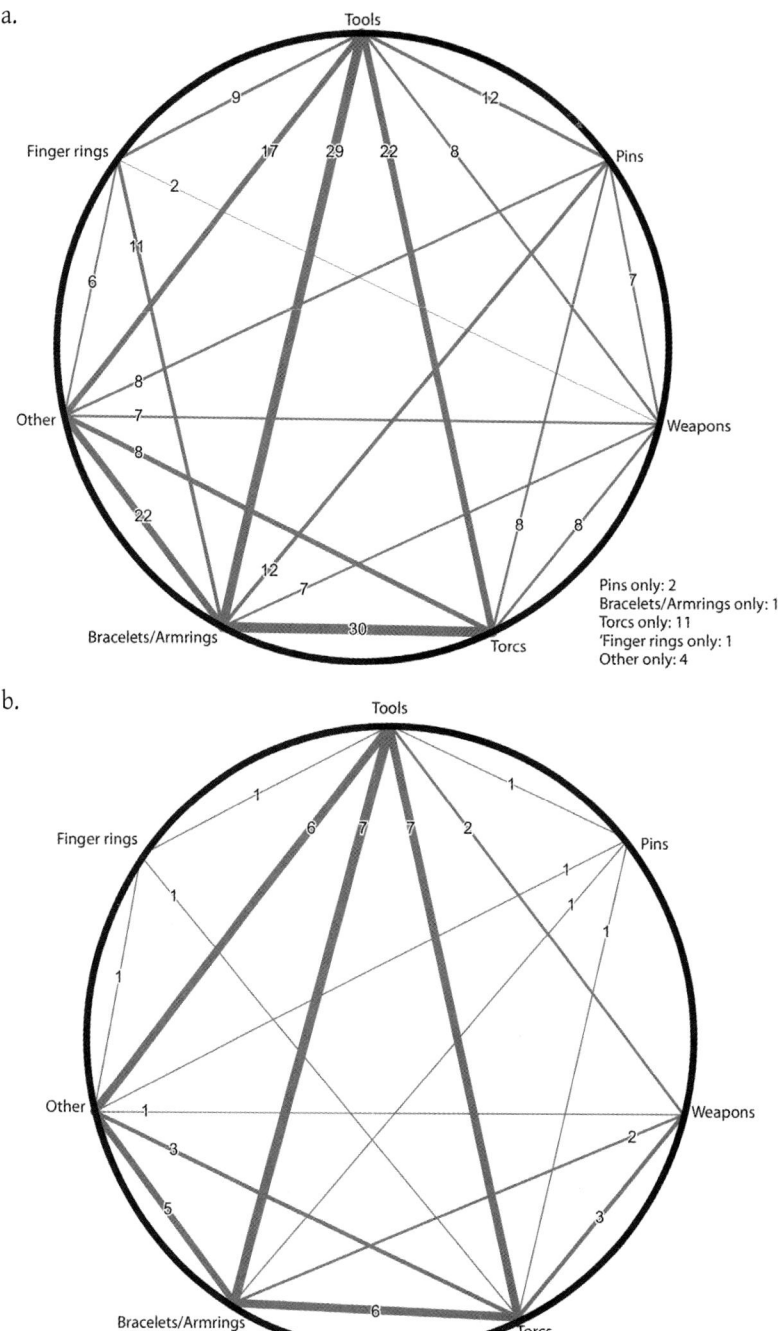

Fig. 2.6: a. Object type connections within 'all types' of ornament hoard (see Appendix 2.1 for details); b. object type connections within 'gold-work only' ornament hoards; c. object type connections within 'mixed' hoards (containing gold-work and copper alloy) (see Appendix 2.1 for details).

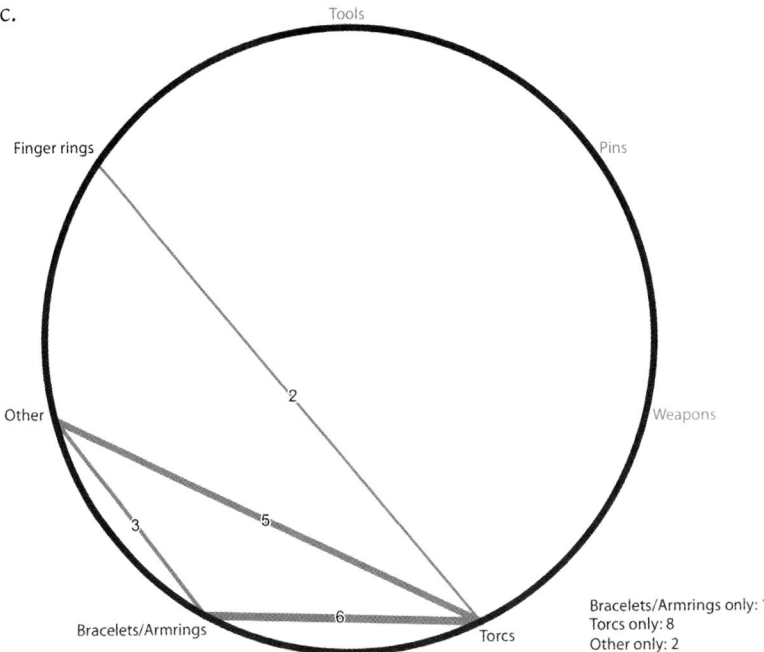

Fig. 2.6: Continued.

geographical dimension to the two clusters: the ST hoards occurring most often in Somerset and Dorset/South Wiltshire and the 'other' hoards in the South Coast region.

Rowlands' clusters overlap significantly in terms of their overall contents, which are actually largely similar except for the presence of spiral-twisted ornaments (Table 2.1). In terms of the 'less' and 'more certain' qualitative categories outlined at the start of this paper, three ST hoards (12.5%) are 'less certain' compared to 21 (c. 50%) of bracelet/armlet hoards. This is in part due to the nature of the deposits, with several 'other' hoards deposited at settlement sites, but also because they include hoards that are poorly recorded and possibly incomplete. Given these overlaps and areas of potential bias, it is best not to draw firm conclusions regarding the existence of a dual-ornament hoard tradition. More compelling are the regional patterns that could correspond with identities and changing fashions, particularly with respect to spiral-twisted ornaments, Sussex Loops and spearhead deposition. The distribution of ST hoards is focussed in the west of southern England while hoards of bracelet/arm-rings (most clearly the Sussex Loop hoards) are concentrated in the east. Whether this relates to chronological and/or social factors is a moot point and the small but notable instances of overlaps between the two groupings suggests that the boundaries between groups were not strictly drawn.

Attempts to identify composition patterns at a national scale should therefore be tempered with awareness of the evidence for very specific, localised connections.

Table 2.1: Ornament types in Rowlands' two hoard 'clusters'

Object type	Spiral twisted group	Other
Spiral-twisted torc	23	–
Spiral-twisted bracelet	4	–
Pin (quoit headed)	7	5
Pin (other)	2	4
Other ornament	7	7
finger-ring	7	8
Torc (ribbon)	1	–
Torc (cast)	2	–
Torc (bar)	1	–
Spiral ring necklace	2	–
Bracelet/armring (annular)	5	10
Bracelet/armring (penannular)	7	5
Bracelet/armring (other)	2	9
Cast, ribbed bracelet	4	2
Sussex Loop	2	8
Tool (palstave)	11	14
Tool (other)	8	7
Weapon (all types)	3	9
Spiral-twisted torc only	3	–
TOTAL no. of hoards	T = 24	T = 42

For instance, two of the largest hoards from Somerset, at Monkswood (Smith 1959b, GB. 42 2(1) and 2(2)) and Taunton Workhouse (*ibid.*, GB. 43 2(1) and 2(2)) contained very similar objects. Similarly, two nearby hoards from Brighton/Lewes (the so called 'Hanley Cross' hoard) (Rowlands 1976, 267) and 'Near Lewes' (Treasure report 2011 T192) both contained combinations of Sussex Loops, a quoit-headed pin and a Tumulus/Urnfield style pin with a disc head and decorated lozenge-shaped plate. These are the only such combinations in the country and both were deposited in unusual ways: the Hanley Cross hoard may in fact have been with a burial (as noted above), while the Near Lewes hoard was contained within a ceramic vessel. These similarities, often in close geographical proximity, relate to particular regional and chronological expressions of identity and fashion situated within larger scale patterning. More work is needed to draw out the full extent of these connections rather than trying to arrive at a one size fits all explanation.

A relatively high proportion (*c.* 28%) of hoards contained an equal number of ornaments and tools/weapons (Table 2.2). In Somerset the pattern is particularly clear and there appears to be a relationship between palstaves and spiral-twisted torcs. Thus the hoards from Weare (Rowlands 1976, 259), Spaxton (*ibid.*, 257–8) and Wedmore

2. Combination, composition and context

Table 2.2: The numerical relationship between ornaments and tools/weapons in hoards containing both ornaments, tools and/or weapons (T = 47)

Number of ornaments relative to tools/weapons	No./(%)
Equal numbers	13 (28%)
±1	7 (13%)
±2	6 (13%)
±3	1 (2%)
±4	3 (7%)
5-9	11 (24%)
10+	6 (13%)

(*ibid.*, 260), comprised of an equal number of spiral-twisted torcs and palstaves. Only in a relatively small number of cases are the number of ornaments and tools greatly out of balance (i.e. by ten or more: Table 2.2), as in the hoards from Gosport (*ibid.*, 239, pl. 56) and Hayling (*ibid.*, 239, pls. 55–6), from close to one another in Hampshire. In both cases palstaves were associated with a single bracelet/arm-ring. The inverse is true at Brading Marsh, on the Isle of Wight, where multiple bracelet/arm-rings were associated with a single spearhead. The exceptions are therefore sometimes patterned in their own right and may even serve to help 'prove the rule'.

The relationship is not straightforward but the sense of an approximate numerical balance existing between ornaments and tools is evident in a considerable number of hoards. This may relate to the processes by which the objects in the hoard were assembled or it could relate to an intentional message of depositional rituals: a way of expressing and creating balance or imbalance in the symbolic force represented by object types. As noted above, this may have related to male or female associations or to other concepts and spheres of life that the objects came to represent.

Modification, manipulation and 'structured deposition'

The intentional spatial patterning and modification of objects within ornament hoards has been noted in several studies (*e.g.* Barber 2001, 162–4; Roberts 2007, 146–7), but the extent and significance of these practices have never been fully pursued. Twenty-nine of the hoards (*c.* 30%) contain one or more instance of these treatments. Two key types of treatment can be distinguished: treatment prior to deposition, and structured and intentionally spatially patterned deposits.

Treatments prior to deposition

Among the 16 hoards with evidence for manipulation prior to deposition, the modification and manipulation of the metalwork is represented by six hoards. This treatment was partly related to the malleable qualities of the metal, as all of the objects treated in this fashion were made of gold.

The gold ribbon torc and/or the bracelets from Winterhay Green, Wiltshire, were coiled to make them unusable (Evans 1881, 89; Rowlands 1976, 256). Both flange-twisted gold torcs from Crow Down hoard from Lambourn, West Berkshire, were also coiled (Varndell et al. 2007, 28). The Tier Cross hoard from near Milton Haven contained two wire torcs that Aldhouse-Green and Northover (1996, 43) suggest were worn as a pair of loosely coiled bracelets before their preparation for concealment, which involved straightening out the everted terminals and tight recoiling. The Cwmjenkin hoard from Heyhope in Wales comprised of three ribbon torcs deposited in a tangled ball (Savory 1958). Similarly, the Priddy hoard from Somerset consisted of a tight ball of four bar torcs, a ribbon torc and several bracelets (Minnitt and Payne 2012). The Cirencester hoard from Gloucestershire comprised of 57 objects of gold and five of bronze, a high proportion of which had been chopped, cut or torn into fragments along with a number of tools which, as noted above, may have belonged to a metalworker (Needham 2004, 26–33). Needham (*ibid.*, 30–1) notes that the fragmentation goes beyond the extent required for recycling, and that the process may have had a symbolic role.

The malleable properties of gold mean it was relatively easy to distort, but the act of manipulating and depositing the material requires attention, particularly as it could have been remelted and recycled. The most prosaic explanation is that these objects were no longer required and were prepared for recycling that did not occur. However, even in the case of the Cirencester hoard, entirely functional explanations may be insufficient. It is more likely that objects were distorted in the course of ritualised practises, in order to symbolically kill them and place them beyond the world of the living (Nebelsick 2000).

A number of 'copper-alloy only' hoards also contain objects that may have been broken through use (e.g. Taunton Workhouse, Somerset: Smith 1959b, GB. 43 2(1) and 2(2)). These were not fine, unused objects, selected for intentional, symbolic deposition. It is possible that at least some were buried with no associated rituals or symbolism and with the intention of recovery, remelting and reworking. In other hoards, most of the objects are in a better condition and some objects appear to have been intentionally broken (e.g. the torcs from Wylye, Wiltshire: Treasure report 2012 T768). There is a danger of imposing a monolithic or dualistic interpretation of hoards based on either functional or symbolic readings of breakage and wear. The best way to assess the original intention of deposition is with respect to patterning in composition and deposition, with each hoard assessed on its own merits as part of the wider phenomenon.

Threading and looping

Ten hoards were manipulated by being threaded, looped or tied onto other objects. In the case of the Norton Fitzwarren hoard (Needham in Ellis 1989), some or all of the eight bracelets/arm-rings appeared to have been tied together prior to deposition. The hoard from Edington Burtle, Somerset, included a lozenge-sectioned bracelet with two attached rings, one looped over the bracelet and another attached only to the other ring (Smith 1959b, GB.44 2(2)). The Monkswood hoard, Somerset, also contained two lozenge-sectioned bracelets looped over one another (*ibid.*, GB. 42 2(1)). The hoard from South Wonston, Hampshire, contained a lozenge-sectioned bracelet with two smaller rings of spiral-twisted rod looped over it (Hughes and Champion 1982).

The Wylye hoard, Wiltshire, contained two examples of spiral-twisted bracelets/arm-rings looped onto spiral-twisted torcs (Treasure report 2012 T786). It also included a spiral-twisted torc with a small ring wrapped around it and a second spiral-twisted torc onto which three finger-rings had been threaded. The latter is particularly notable as the spiral-twisted torc from the Hollingbury hoard, Sussex, also carried three threaded finger-rings (*Arch. J.* 1848; Rowlands 1976, 143).

The threading of rings onto other objects is also a feature of gold ornaments of the Penard phase. In the case of the Haxey hoard, Lincolnshire, three gold rings were threaded onto a large flange-twisted torc (Eogan 1967, 149). The size of the torc suggests that it could also have fitted around the waist as well as the neck. An unusual untwisted, plain section on one side of the torc may have been intentionally designed with the display of rings in mind, in which case threading was an integral feature of the original design rather than a later addition. The bracelet from Grunty Fen, Cambridgeshire, had six threaded rings (*ibid.*, 141–3), while the bracelet from Widsor, Berkshire, had five threaded rings (Treasure report 2009 T755), and the coiled twisted gold torc from northeast Norfolk had nine threaded rings (Varndell 2004).

The threading and looping of rings or finger-rings is therefore a notable feature shared by both Penard and Taunton phases of ornament hoard deposition. All but five of the six threaded finger-rings occurred in groups of three or multiples of three. If this was an intentional practice, and more examples are required, then it suggests a close connection between practices in the two phases. It is likely that some of these instances of looping and threading occurred shortly prior to deposition, possibly as a way of keeping broken lengths of ornament together prior to anticipated episodes of recycling. In other cases it may have been a feature of how the ornaments were actually worn or part of the collection process prior to deposition.

While the number of rings may also have been important, if they were a feature of the ornaments as worn in life, they may have been related to the successful achievement of stages of life and rites of passage. However, if undertaken for the depositional act itself (as some of the looping of bracelets and torcs appear to have been), it may have substituted for human digits and limbs. This is of note because the non-funerary deposition of ornament hoards meant that they lacked the structure of a body on which the objects could be seen, displayed and interpreted.

Nesting, vertical distinctions and stacking

Thirteen hoards include the nesting or stacking of ornaments within deposits, including both hoards of copper-alloy and gold ornaments. Within the gold hoard from Towednack, Cornwall, a small flange-twisted torc had been placed within a larger torc of the same type and four penannular bracelets in different states of completion and two gold rods were 'neatly arranged' within them (Hawkes 1932, 177–86; Eogan 1967, 144). The workmen who discovered the goldwork hoard at Capel Isaf, Powys, also reported that a ribbon torc and four bracelet/armlets had been deposited in a 'tight mass', 'wrapped round each other', placed under a large glacial erratic slab (Savory 1977, 37–63). Similarly, and also from Powys, in the Maesmelan hoard a larger bracelet had been placed around a smaller bracelet (Green et al. 1983). At Binstead, West Sussex, a pair of rings (in the form miniature bracelets) had their hooked terminals interlinked (Varndell 1998/9, 10–11).

In the copper-alloy hoard from Spaxton in the Quantock Hills, Somerset, two twisted torcs, were found, 'one lying on the other', with a palstave set in the centre of each torc (Harford 1803, 94; Rowlands 1976, 257–8). The nesting of a palstave within a spiral-twisted torc was also a feature of the aforementioned hoard from Hollingbury, Sussex (*Arch. J.* 1848; Rowlands 1976, 143). The vertical spatial arrangement seen in the case of the Spaxton hoard is also found in the Grunty Fen hoard, Cambridgeshire, where there was *c.* 30cm of peat between the gold flange-twisted torc and the copper-alloy palstaves, with the torc being at the bottom, and the deposits possibly separated by a sod of peat (Eogan 1967, 140–1). In the hoard from Llanwrthwl, Powys, Wales, two gold flange-twisted torcs were found below a large stone and a heap of smaller stones, and beneath the torcs was a small stone overlying two more torcs (Savory 1958, 52–4, pls. i–ii; Eogan 1967, 153–4, pls. 18–19). Furthermore, a hoard consisting of a single complete bracelet and 21 fragmentary ring or bracelet fragments on the Isle of Wight, the bracelet/ring fragments were found just below the top soil and were stacked above the complete bracelet (Treasure report 2012 T430). Finally, the hoard from Church Farm, Ripple, consisted of a series of bracelets deposited as a group in the centre of the pit, with each bracelet intentionally stacked one on top of the other, with a finger-ring placed in the centre (Parfitt n.d.; O'Connor n.d.). The bracelets were graded by weight and by size, with the heaviest bracelet with the largest internal diameter placed on the bottom of the stack.

The practice of nesting ornaments tightly over one another may have been related to their safekeeping and storage but, given its prevalence and the evidence for threading and looping reviewed above, it can also be interpreted as a way of associating different object types (i.e. torcs and palstaves), and the symbolic principles they may have represented. As in the case of threading and looping, by physically wrapping objects around others, they were re-animated, perhaps with reference to the bodies that were absent. Indeed, the stacking and grading of the bracelet/arm-rings from Church Farm, Ripple, with centrally placed finger-rings may even have evoked an absent limb.

The horizontal and vertical distinctions noted above are suggestive of care and structure in deposition and probably related to the structured ritual practices in which they were laid down. The distance between certain object and material types may have related to and communicated their different symbolic significance. For instance, the copper-alloy palstaves and gold flange-twisted torc were separated in the Grunty Fen hoard (Eogan 1967, 140–1), possibly on the grounds of material and object type, while among the Isle of Wight (Treasure report 2012 T430) and Towednack hoards, objects were seemingly separated on the basis of completeness.

Complex spatial arrangements

More complex spatial patterning occurs within seven hoards. At Gosport, Hampshire, 18 palstaves were found set vertically in the ground, blade downward, accompanied by a single bracelet/arm-ring (Rowlands 1976, 239, pl. 56). At South Dumpton Down, Kent four palstaves with unsharpened blades were placed together on their side and arranged in an arc or fan arrangement (Barber 2001, 163). Overlying the palstaves was a slab of tabular flint and higher in the fill of the pit a palstave was found lying on its face, with a bronze bracelet resting on top of it (*ibid.*). The Brading Marsh hoard consisted of eleven bracelet/arm-rings and a spearhead. The finder reported that the armlets were 'linked together, surrounding the spear[head]' (Roach Smith 1882, 423–4; Rowlands 1976, 238). The Gosport, South Dumpton and Brading Marsh hoards involved very particular practices in which objects are set in contrast both spatially and in terms of their function and number.

The Hollingbury hoard was apparently found under a mound and the finder reported that the four Sussex Loops were arranged as the points of a square, with a spiral-twisted torc within them and (as noted above) three finger-rings threaded onto its length. Within the torc a broken palstave had been placed, its blade positioned between the terminal ends (Fig. 2.7; *Arch. J.* 1848, 324–5). As in case of threading, looping and nesting, the Hollingbury hoard can be related to notion of incorporeal substitutes for bodies and limbs: here the torc 'wears' the finger-rings while the positioning of the palstave evokes the neck and head and the pairing and separation of Sussex Loop bracelet/arm-rings are arranged as if worn by four absent limbs.

In the case of the aforementioned hoard from Wylye, Wiltshire, spatial patterning took the form of deposition in two separate pits, a few meters apart (Treasure report 2012 T786). Within the respective deposits, similarities in type and decoration can be identified but differences can be identified in terms of weight and size of the objects. The objects were found in 'deposit 1' and the heaviest in 'deposit 2', including two 'oversized' torcs and the massive quoit-headed pin. It may also be noted that in the case of the hoard from Tiers Cross, Pembrokeshire, the finds were apparently made in three separate find-spots spread out over 500m or less in a straight line, although archaeological fieldwork undertaken was unable to verify the claim (Aldhouse-Green and Northover 1996, 42). The splitting of deposits into separate pits may have served the same function as other vertical and horizontal distinctions noted above: to compare and contrast properties and symbolic principles. The Wylye deposits may even relate to notions of scale and size and possibly – given the scale of the torcs

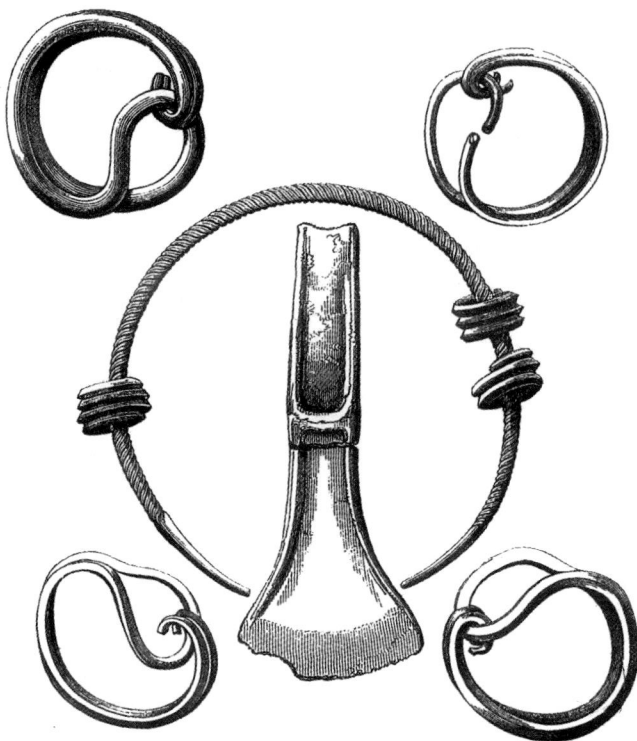

Fig. 2.7: The reported spatial relationships between the objects found within the Hollingbury Hoard, Sussex (after Arch. J. 1848).

and presence of palstaves in 'deposit 1' – a male (deposit 1) and female (deposit 2) distinction.

Special deposits within domestic contexts

A number of ornament hoards have been found within domestic buildings and structures (e.g. Chalton, Hampshire: Cunliffe 1970; Black Patch, Sussex: Drewett 1982; Dumpton Down, Kent: Barber 2001, 163). At Bestwall Quarry, House 1, two bracelets appear to have been separate closing deposits within a roundhouse (Ladle and Woodward 2009, 72, 272, 275, 368–9, figs. 47, 184). One was deposited approximately above the position of the former hearth, the other at the base of the pit associated with the burnt mound; the deposits lay on a line that defined the axis of the house (taken as a line through the centre of the doorway) (*ibid.*, fig. 47), and therefore do not qualify as a hoard in the traditional sense defined above. The association between ornaments and settlement is of note given their rarity in funerary contexts. It reinforces the apparent conceptual separation between metalwork and the dead but also (given the prominence of 'tools' in ornament hoards) suggests that there was willingness to associate functional and non-functional metalwork in the same hoard deposits.

Discussion and conclusions

A number of regional and supra-regional patterns have been observed in the preceding study. Ornaments designed for different parts of the body were made in different ways, with little room for diversion from normative patterns that applied across southern England and beyond. On the other hand, objects such as Sussex Loops represent a very particular regional expression of fashion, identity or depositional practice. Furthermore, different object combinations and hoard compositions were in use for copper-alloy and goldwork hoards (*cf.* Roberts 2007). It remains to be demonstrated (through more absolute dating evidence) whether this related to a chronological change, but it certainly had a geographical dimension, with goldwork hoards falling out with the main concentrations of copper-alloy hoards (Fig. 2.2). It can also be related to social and ritual categories and concepts that governed where particular materials and objects could be deposited and to the expression of regional identities.

Some hoards could have been intended for retrieval but the evidence for structured deposition, non-functional manipulation and the balancing of tools and ornaments presented above, suggests that many (if not all) were deposited in the course of ritualised practices and were not intended for retrieval (*cf.* Dietrich 2014). The preference for palstaves over other tool and weapon types (especially contemporary dirks and rapiers) was noted above and their meaning may have been informed with reference to ornaments and the household sphere. It was possible to identify combinations and sets of objects, a feature that connects them to contemporary Continental European costumes (*cf.* Wels-Weyrauch 1989) and suggests that (at least some) ornaments were intended to be coordinated when worn. The looping and threading of objects onto others in hoards may have evoked absent limbs and bodies despite their separation from bodies in funerary contexts. Many of the objects from ornament hoards were in a fragmentary condition, some worn out through use or for recycling, others perhaps symbolically broken or killed, these objects were perhaps passed from the land of living into a supernatural Otherworld in which concepts of non-corporeal bodies may have been relevant.

The southern English hoards thus present some important contradictions: the combination of regional and supra-regional patterns, and the combination of traits of individual dress and bodies with the more communal and anonymous character of hoard deposits. To understand why these attitudes changed it is important to set ornament hoards in a wider context of contemporary social, economic and ritual practices. Bradley (2007, 197–9) has noted the existence of strong connections between Middle Bronze Age settlements and cemeteries, with a wider range and greater proportion of people receiving burials than during the Early Bronze Age. Although this pattern has some regional manifestations, it appears remarkably consistent across the country (*ibid.*). Bradley (*ibid.*, 201) suggests that objects that signalled social elites may have been removed prior to cremation and deposited in hoards and in watery locations. The transformation of funerary and depositional practices appears to reflect a fundamental shift in the way communities could communicate with the Otherworld.

During the Early Bronze Age, the relatively small proportion of the dead who received formal burial were equipped with grave goods that included ornaments and other finery appear to have acted as idealised or selected representatives of the living community (Thomas 1991; Traherne 1995; Garwood 2011). The separation of the deposition of objects and bodies suggests new strategies for communicating with the Otherworld. However, the evocation of bodies by means of looping, nesting and spatial structure within hoard deposits may represent a continuation and development of Early Bronze Age funerary practices: dressing absent, perhaps idealised or ancestral bodies without the need for the corporeal remains of particular individuals to be present.

In order to explain why the distribution of ornaments and ornament hoards are so restricted, primarily to southern England, the contemporary social and economic context is important. The South of England has produced the vast majority of the contemporary evidence for co-axial field systems and agricultural intensification in Britain (Yates 2007). The ability to produce and ritually deposit ornaments and dress accessories may therefore be seen as a product of this regime of agricultural intensification. Agricultural surpluses can provide the means of acquiring status related metalwork and enclosure, as Yates notes, is strongly associated with 'power and prestige' (ibid., 121), and indeed with 'keeping up appearances' in the form of high-status objects and dress accessories (ibid., 127). Despite the unprecedented agricultural intensification in this part of the country, there was no socio-economic aggrandisement in the form of clear evidence for more complex social structure or settlement nucleation (Bradley 2007, 187–202). This situation may have been partly related to the regularity with which high-status metalwork was deposited in the same regions as field systems appeared (Yates 2007, Ch. 12, *in passim*, especially 121–2, 127–9).

A socio-political model for the southern distribution of ornament hoards is also suggested by the intensity of cross-Channel trade during the Middle Bronze Age (O'Connor 1980). It may have been important that individuals in this region share the same dress and ornament fashions; even if they were deposited differently (*cf.* Needham 2000). Ornament hoards may thus have provided a way of dealing with material that had to be accepted due to socio-political forces but which was at odds with existing ritual practices connected to the deposition of bodies and the construction of identities for the dead across Britain as a whole.

In discussing Bronze Age hoards of the southern Netherlands, Fontijn (2002, 239) has noted that ornaments and dress accessories have a referential rather than a practical role, signalling social status and roles in a way that weapons and tools do not. The use of ornaments to adorn the dead serves to construct identities, while their placement in hoards may deconstruct those identities (*ibid.*). The inclusion of tools in the same hoards and the evidence for fragmentation and intentional breakage serves to reinforce this point for the Middle Bronze Age hoards of southern England. Fontijn (*ibid.*) argues that the deposition of bodily ornament and dress accessories can be used as a way of dealing with personal identities that, for ritual and socio-political reasons, should be temporary, ambiguous or related to special roles. In southern

England during the Middle Bronze Age, deposition may have taken place in order to maintain the socio-political and ritual *status quo* during a period and region of agricultural intensification (*cf.* Yates 2007, Ch. 12). Thus the sacrifice of ornaments in hoard deposits may have served (intentionally or indirectly) to keep the region broadly similar to the rest of the country in terms of social hierarchies and settlement nucleation. The symbolism and significance of ornament and dress accessory hoards can thus be addressed in a more holistic fashion when linked to economic and socio-political factors that played out at regional and supra-regional scales.

Note
1. For details of Treasure reports cited in this paper see https://finds.org.uk/.

Bibliography
Adams, K. (2013) GLO-6535E4, A Bronze Age hoard. Webpage available at: http://finds.org.uk/database/artefacts/record/id/570863 [accessed March 2016].
Aldhouse-Green, S. and Northover, J. P. (1996) Recent finds of Late Bronze Age Gold from Wales. *Antiquaries Journal* 76, 223–28.
Anderson, J. (1883) Notice of urns in the museum that have been found with articles of use or ornament. *Proceedings of the Society of Antiquaries of Scotland* 17, 446–59.
Anderson, J. (1884) Notice of the gold ornaments found at Lower Largo, and of the silver ornaments etc found at Norrie's Law, near Largo, recently presented to the museum by Robert Dundas, esq. of Arniston. *Proceedings of the Society of Antiquaries of Scotland* 18, 233–47.
Annable, F. K. and Simpson, D. D. A. (1964) *Guide Catalogue of the Neolithic and Bronze Age Collections in Devizes Museum*. Devizes, Wiltshire Archaeological and Natural History Society at the Museum.
Antiq. J. (1926) Bronze Age hoard from Sussex. *Antiquaries Journal* 6, 444–6.
Arch. J. (1848) Archaeological intelligence. *Archaeological Journal* 5, 322–37.
Arch. J. (1849) Proceedings of the meetings of the Archaeological Institute. *Archaeological Journal* 6, 81.
Arch. J. (1850) Proceedings at the meetings of the Archaeological Institute *Archaeological Journal* 7, 64–90.
Arch. J. (1873) Proceedings at the meetings of the Royal Archaeological Institute. *Archaeological Journal* 30, 90–101.
Arch. J. (1880) Antiquities and works of art exhibited. *Archaeological Journal* 37, 107.
Barber, M. (2001) A time and a place for bronze. In J. Brück (ed.) *Bronze Age Landscapes: Tradition and Transformation*, 161–9. Oxford, Oxbow Books.
Basford, F. (2012) IOW-B3F7D1, a Bronze Age hoard. Webpage available at: http://finds.org.uk/database/artefacts/record/id/505864 [accessed March 2016].
Bergerbrant, S. (2007) *Bronze Age Identities: Costume, Conflict and Contact in Northern Europe 1600-1300 BC*. Lindome, Bricoleur Press.
Bergerbrant, S., Bender Jørgensen, L. and Fossøy, S. H. (2013) Appearance in Bronze Age Scandinavia as seen from the Nybøl burial. *European Journal of Archaeology* 16(2), 247–67.
Bradley, R. (2007) *The Prehistory of Britain and Ireland*. Cambridge, Cambridge University Press.
Bradley, R. (2013) Hoards and the deposition of metalwork. In H. Fokkens and A. Harding (eds.) *Handbook of the European Bronze Age*. Oxford, Oxford University Press.
Burgess, C. B. (1980) *The Age of Stonehenge*. London, Dent.
Burgess, C. B. and Gerloff, S. (1981) *The Dirks and Rapiers of Great Britain and Ireland*. Munich, Beck (*Prahistorische Bronzefunde*, IV/7).

Byard, A. (2009) BERK-A5FFE5, a Bronze Age bracelet. Webpage available at: http://finds.org.uk/database/artefacts/record/id/281365 [accessed March 2016].

Chapman, J. (2000) *Fragmentation in Archaeology: People, Places and Broken Objects in the Prehistory of South-Eastern Europe*. London, Routledge.

Callander, J. G. (1921) A Bronze Age hoard from Glen Trool, Stewartry of Kirkcudbright. *Proceedings of the Society of Antiquaries of Scotland* 55, 29–37.

Coles, J. (1963) The Hilton (Dorset) gold ornaments. *Antiquity* 36, 132–3.

Coles, J. (1964) Scottish Middle Bronze Age metalwork. *Proceedings of the Society of Antiquaries of Scotland* 97, 82–156.

Colt Hoare, R. (1812) *The Ancient History of Wiltshire*. London, William Miller.

Combe, B. H. (1863) Gold found at Mountfield. *Sussex Archaeological Collections* 15, 238–40.

Crawford, O. G. S. and Wheeler, R. E. M. (1921) The Llynfawr and other hoards of the Bronze Age. *Archaeologia* 71, 133–40.

Cunliffe, B. (1970) A Bronze Age settlement at Chalton Hants (Site 78). *Antiquaries Journal* 50, 1–13.

Dietrich, O. (2014) Learning from 'scrap' about Late Bronze Age hoarding practices: a biographical approach to individual acts of dedication in large metal hoards of the Carpathian Basin. *European Journal of Archaeology* 17(3), 468–86.

Dietrich, O. and Mörtz, T. (forthcoming) Sockets full of scrap? Remarks on deliberate fragmentation in Late Bronze Age metal deposits in south-eastern and north-western Europe. In A. Blanco-González and J. C. Chapman, (eds.) *Deliberate Fragmentation Revisited. Assessing Social and Material Agency in the Archaeological Record. Proceedings of a session held at the 19th Annual Meeting of the European Association of Archaeologists in Pilsen, 7th September 2013*.

Dixon, F. (1849) On bronze or brass relics, celts etc found in Sussex. *Sussex Archaeological Collections* 2, 260–9.

Drew, C. D. (1934) Bronze Age hoard from Haselbury Bryan. *Proceedings of the Dorset Natural History and Archaeological Society* 56, 131–2.

Drewett, S. (1982) Later Bronze Age downland economy and excavations at Black Patch, East Sussex. *Proceedings of the Prehistoric Society* 48, 321–400.

Ellis, P. (1989) Norton Fitzwarren hillfort: a report on the excavation by Nancy and Philip Langmaid between 1968 and 1971. *Somerset Archaeology and Natural History* 133, 1–74.

Eogan, G. (1967) The associated finds of gold bar torcs. *Journal of the Royal Society of Antiquaries of Ireland* 98(2), 129–75.

Eogan, G. (1983) Ribbon torcs in Britain and Ireland. In D. V. Clarke and A. O'Connor (eds.) *From the Stone Age to the 'Forty-Five: Studies Presented to R. B. K. Stevenson*, 87–126. Edinburgh, John Donald.

Eogan, G. (1994) *The Accomplished Art*. Oxford, Oxbow (Oxbow Monograph 42).

Evans, J. (1881) *The Ancient Bronze Implements, Weapons, and Ornaments of Great Britain and Ireland*. London, Longmans, Green, and Co.

Fontijn, D. R. (2002) *Sacrificial Landscapes. Cultural Biographies of Persons, Objects and 'Natural' Places in the Bronze Age of the Southern Netherlands*. Leiden, University of Leiden.

Franks, A. W. (1864) Three fragments of gold from Mountfield, near Battle. *Proceedings of the Society of Antiquaries of London* 2 (2nd Series), 247–8.

Garrow, D. and Gosden, C. (2012) *Technologies of Enchantment? Exploring Celtic Art: 400 BC to AD 100*. Oxford, Oxford University Press.

Garwood, P. (2011) Making the dead. In G. Hey, P. Garwood, M. Robinson, A. Barclay and P. Bradley (eds.) *The Thames Through Time: Volume 1, Section 2; Earlier Prehistory*, 383–432. Oxford, Oxford Archaeology.

Green, H. S., Guilbert, G. and Cowell, M. (1983) Two gold bracelets from Maesmelan Farm Powys. *Bulletin of the Board of Celtic Studies* 30(3–4), 394–8.

Gwilt, A., Lodwick, M., and Davis, M. (2004) Burton, Wrexham: Middle Bronze Age hoard of gold adornments and bronze tool with a pot (04.2). *Treasure Annual Report* 2004, 198–9.

Harford, C. J. (1803) An account of some antiquities discovered on the Quantock Hills, in Somersetshire, in the year 1794. *Archaeologia* 14, 94–8.

Harris, S. (2012) From the parochial to the universal: comparing cloth cultures in the Bronze Age. *European Journal of Archaeology* 15(1), 61–97.

Hawkes, C. F. C. (1932) The Towednack gold hoard. *Man* 32, 222–39.

Hawkes, C. F. C. (1942) The Deverel Urn and the Picardy Pin: a phase of Bronze Age settlement in Kent. *Proceedings of the Prehistoric Society* 3, 26–47.

Hinds, K. (2013) HAMP-1AE583, a Bronze Age hoard. Webpage available at: http://finds.org.uk/database/artefacts/record/id/565606 [accessed March 2016].

Holleyman, G. A. (1948) Brighton Loops and flint implements from Falmer Hill. *Sussex Notes and Queries* 11, 60–1.

Hughes, M. and Champion, T. (1982) A Middle Bronze Age ornament hoard from South Wonston, Hampshire. *Proceedings of the Prehistoric Society* 48, 487–9.

Huson, S. (1999) A find of Middle Bronze Age bracelets from Cranleigh. *Surrey Archaeological Collections* 86, 203–5.

JBAA (1865) Proceedings of the Association. *Journal of the British Archaeological Association* 11, 232.

Kenny, J. (1993) Lavant: the reservoir site at Chalkpit Lane. In Chichester Excavations Committee (ed.) *The Archaeology of Chichester and District*, 26–30. Chichester, Chichester Excavations Committee.

Knight, M. G., Ormrod, T. and Pearce, S. (2015) *The Bronze Age Metalwork of South Western Britain. A Corpus of Material Found Between 1983 and 2014*. Oxford, Archaeopress (British Archaeological Reports, British Series, 610).

Ladle, L. and Woodward, A. (2009) *Excavations at Bestwall Quarry, Wareham, 1992-2005, Volume 1: The Prehistoric Landscape*. Dorchester, Dorset Natural History and Archaeological Society (Dorset Natural History and Archaeological Society Monograph 19).

Lawson, A. (1979) Two quoit-headed pins in the British Museum. *Antiquaries Journal* 59(1), 121–4.

Manley, J. and White, S. (1996) A very long quoit-headed pin and a decorated annular armring from the Newhaven area, East Sussex. *Sussex Archaeological Collections* 134, 233–5.

Minter, F. (2002) SF9909, a Bronze Age pin. Webpage available at: http://finds.org.uk/database/artefacts/record/id/33509 [accessed March 2016].

Minnitt, S. and Payne, N. (2012) A hoard of Middle Bronze Age gold ornaments from Priddy, Somerset. In J. R. Trigg (ed.) *Of Things Gone but not Forgotten. Essays in Archaeology for Joan Taylor*, 109–14. Oxford, Archaeopress (British Archaeological Reports, International Series 2434).

Nebelsick, L. (2000) "Rent asunder": ritual violence in Late Bronze Age hoards. In C. Pare (ed.) *Metals Make the World Go Round*, 160–75. Oxford, Oxbow Books.

Needham, S. (1990) The Penard-Wilburton succession: new metalwork finds from Croxton (Norfolk) and Thirsk (Yorkshire). *Antiquaries Journal* 70(2), 253–70.

Needham, S. (1996) Chronology and periodisation in the British Bronze Age. *Acta Archaeologica* 67, 121–40.

Needham, S. (2000) Power pulses across a cultural divide: cosmologically driven exchange between Armorica and Wessex. *Proceedings of the Prehistoric Society* 66, 151–207.

Needham, S. (2001) Cantley, South Yorkshire: gold torc (1), Middle Bronze Age bronze spearhead fragment (2) and bronze instrument (3) (2001 T43). *Treasure Annual Report 2001*, 16.

Needham, S. (2004) Cirencester area, Gloucestershire: Bronze Age gold and base-metal scatter (2004 T416). *Treasure Annual Report 2004*, 26–33.

Needham, S. (2005) Transforming Beaker Culture in North-West Europe: processes of fusion and fission. *Proceedings of the Prehistoric Society* 71, 171–217.

Needham, S., Parham, D., and Frieman, C. (eds.) (2013) *Claimed by the Sea: Salcombe, Langdon Bay and other Marine Finds of the Bronze Age*. York, Council for British Archaeology (Council for British Archaeology Research Report 173).

Needham, S., Parker Pearson, M., Tyler, A., Richards, M., and Jay, M. (2010) A first 'Wessex 1' date from Wessex. *Antiquity* 84, 363–73.

Norfolk Museums Service (1977) *Bronze Age Metalwork in Norwich Castle Museum*. Norwich, Norfolk Museums Service.

O'Connor, B. (1980) *Cross Channel Relations in the Later Bronze Age*. Oxford, British Archaeological Reports (British Archaeological Reports, International Series 91).

O'Connor, B. (1989) The Middle Bronze Age of southern England. In *Dynamique du Bronze Moyen en Europe Occidentale, Strasbourg: Actes du 113e Congres national des Sociétés savants*, 515–21. Paris, Comité des travaux historiques et scientifiques.

O'Connor, B. (1991) Bronze Age metalwork from Cranborne Chase: a catalogue. In J. Barrett, R. Bradley and M. Hall (eds) *Papers on the Prehistoric Archaeology of Cranborne Chase*, 231–41. Oxford, Oxbow Books.

O'Connor, B. (n.d.) Church Farm hoard, Ripple. Unpublished report, Department of Britain, Europe and Prehistory, British Museum archive.

Parfitt, K. (n.d.) A Middle Bronze Age ornament hoard from Ripple, near Deal. Unpublished report, Department of Britain, Europe and Prehistory, British Museum archive.

Parfitt, K. (1994) A possible Bronze Age grave at Walmer 1910. *Kent Archaeological Review* 116, 133–5.

Payne, N. (2007) SOM-1C2C53, a Bronze Age hoard. Webpage available at: http://finds.org.uk/database/artefacts/record/id/189967 [accessed March 2016].

Pearce, S. M. (1983) *The Bronze Age Metalwork of South Western Britain*. Oxford, British Archaeological Reports (British Series 120).

PDNHAS (1964) Recent discoveries and accessions. *Proceedings of the Dorset Natural History and Archaeological Society* 86, 115.

Pearce, S. M. and Padley, T. (1977) The Bronze Age find from Tredarvah, Penzance. *Cornish Archaeology* 16, 25–41.

Piggott, C. M. (1949) A Late Bronze Age hoard from Blackrock in Sussex and its significance. *Proceedings of the Prehistoric Society* 15, 107–21.

Pring, J. H. (1880) On some evidences of the occupation of the ancient site of Taunton by the Britons. *Archaeological Journal* 37, 94–8.

PSAL (1901) Thursday June 20th 1901. *Proceedings of the Society of Antiquaries of London* 1901, 388–412.

Randsborg, K. and Christensen, K. (2006) *Bronze Age Oak-Coffin Graves: Archaeology and Dendro-Dating*. Copenhagen, Blackwell-Munksgaard (Acta Archaeologica 77).

Richards, C. and Thomas, J. (1984) Ritual activity and structured deposition in Neolithic Wessex. In R. Bradley and J. Gardiner (eds.) *Neolithic Studies: A Review of Some Current Research*, 189–218. Oxford, British Archaeological Reports (British Archaeological Reports, British Series 133).

Roach Smith, C. (1874) Gold torques and armillae discovered in Kent. *Archaeologia Cantiana* 9, 1–11.

Roach Smith, C. (1882) A hoard of bronze bracelets at Brading, I. W. *Journal of the British Archaeological Association* 38, 423–4.

Roberts, B. (2007) Adorning the living but not the dead: a reassessment of Middle Bronze Age ornaments in Britain. *Proceedings of the Prehistoric Society* 73, 135–67.

Roberts, B., Uckelmann, M., and Brandherm, D. (2013) Old Father Time: the Bronze Age chronology of Western Europe. In H. Fokkens and A. Harding (eds.) *The Oxford Handbook of the European Bronze Age*, 17–46. Oxford, Oxford University Press.

Rohl, B. and Needham, S. (1998) *The Circulation of Metal in the British Bronze Age: the Application of Lead Isotope Analysis*. London, British Museum (British Museum Occasional Paper 102).

Rowlands, M. J. (1971) A group of incised decoration armrings and their significance for the Middle Bronze Age of southern Britain. *British Museum Quarterly* 35 (Nos. 1–4), 183–99.

Rowlands, M. J. (1976) *The Production and Distribution of Metalwork in the Middle Bronze Age in Southern Britain*. Oxford, British Archaeological Reports (British Archaeological Reports, British Series 32).

Savory, H. (1958) The Late Bronze Age in Wales: some new discoveries and new interpretations. *Archaeologica Cambrensis* 107, 3–63.

Savory, H. (1977) A new hoard of Bronze Age gold ornaments from [Capel Isaf, Dyfed] Wales. *Archaeol Atlantica* 2, 37–53.

Sheridan, A. (2007) Dating the Scottish Bronze Age: 'There is clearly much that the material can still tell us'. In C. Burgess P. Topping and F. M. Lynch (eds.), *Beyond Stonehenge: Essays on the Bronze Age in honour of Colin Burgess*, 162–85. Oxford, Oxbow Books.

Smith, M. A. (1959a) Some Somerset hoards and their place in the Bronze Age of southern Britain. *Proceedings of the Prehistoric Society* 25, 144–87.

Smith, M. A. (1959b) Middle Bronze Age Hoards from southern England. *Inv. Arch Great Britain* 7, 42–7.

Smith, S. (2011) SUSS-C5D042, a Bronze Age hoard. Webpage available at: http://finds.org.uk/database/artefacts/record/id/437360 [accessed March 2016].

Sørensen, M. L. S. (1997) Reading dress: the construction of social categories and identities in Bronze Age Europe. *Journal of European Archaeology* 5(1), 93–114.

Sørensen, M. L. S. (2013) Identity, gender, and dress in the European Bronze Age. In H. Fokkens and A. Harding (eds.) *The Oxford Handbook of the European Bronze Age*, 216–33. Oxford, Oxford University Press.

Stradling, W. (1854) A young turf-bearer's find in the Turbaries. *Proceedings of the Somersetshire Archaeological and Natural History Society* 1854, 91–4.

Taylor, J. (1980) *Bronze Age Goldwork of the British Isles*. Cambridge, Cambridge University Press.

Taylor, R. J. (1982) The hoard from West Buckland, Somerset. *Antiquaries Journal* 62, 13–17.

Thomas, J. (1991) Reading the body: beaker funerary practices in Britain In P. Garwood, F. Jenning, R. Skeates and J. Toms (eds.) *Sacred and Profane: proceedings of a conference on archaeology, ritual and religion, Oxford 1989*, 33–42. Oxford, Oxford University Committee for Archaeology (Oxford University Committee for Archaeology Monographs 32).

Traherne, P. (1995) The warrior's beauty: the masculine body and self-identity in Bronze-Age Europe. *Journal of European Archaeology* 3(1), 105–44.

Tyrrell, R. (2009) BUC-C07E88, a Bronze Age torc. Webpage available at: http://finds.org.uk/database/artefacts/record/id/266606 [accessed March 2016].

Yates, D. T. (2007) *Land, Power and Prestige. Bronze Age Field Systems in Southern England*. Oxbow, Oxbow Books.

Varndell, G. (1998/9) Binstead, West Sussex: two Bronze Age gold rings linked together. *Treasure Annual Report 1998-1999*, 10–11.

Varndell, G. (2004) Lambourn, Berkshire: two Middle Bronze Age armlets and three bracelets (2004 T348). *Treasure Annual Report 2004*, 21.

Varndell, G., Coe, D., Hey, G., and Canti, M. (2007) The Crow Down hoard, Lambourn, West Berkshire. *Oxford Journal of Archaeology* 26(3), 215–329.

Warne, C. 1872. *Ancient Dorset, the Celtic, Roman, Saxon and Danish Antiquities of the County*. Bournemouth, D. Sydenham.

Wels-Weyrauch, U. (1989) Mittelbronzezeitliche Frauentrachten in Süddeutschland. In *Dynamique du Bronze Moyen en Europe Occidentale, Strasbourg: Actes du 113e Congres national des Sociétés savants*, 117–34. Paris, Comité des travaux historiques et scientifiques.

Williams, D. (2013). SUR-B41DB6, a Bronze Age hoard. Webpage available at: http://finds.org.uk/database/artefacts/record/id/560976 [accessed March 2016].

Wilson, D. (1863) *Prehistoric Annals of Scotland*. London, Macmillan.

Appendix 2.1: Middle Bronze Age ornament hoards from Britain

No.	Hoard name	County	References	Comment
England				
1	Crow Down, Lambourn	Berkshire	Varndell et al. 2007	G
2	Sonning	Berkshire	Rowlands 1976, 224, pl. 11 (3)	–
3	Windsor	Berkshire	Byard 2009	G
4	Ellesborough area	Buckinghamshire	Tyrrell 2009	G
5	Granta (Grunty) Fen, Stretham	Cambridgeshire	Eogan 1967, 141–3	M
6	Grunty Fen	Cambridgeshire	Eogan 1967, 140–1	M
7	Hampton	Cheshire	Eogan 1967, 143	G
8	Towednack	Cornwall	Hawkes 1932, 177–86	G
9	Tredarvah, Penzance	Cornwall	Pearce and Padley 1977	L
10	Salcombe	Devon	Needham et al. 2013, 86; Knight et al. 2015, 44, no. 163	L
11	Bryanston, Near Blandford	Dorset	British Museum registration book for 1892 (1892, 0901.321–5)	L
12	Eglesham Meadow, Dorchester, Hearth pit	Dorset	Pearce 1983, 469, no. 372	L
13	Grimstone	Dorset	PDNHAS 1964, 115; Rowlands 1976, 232	–
14	Hazelbury Bryan	Dorset	British Museum registration book for 1892 (1892, 0901.326–8); Drew 1934; Rowlands 1976, 232	–
15	Hilton	Dorset	Coles 1963, 132–3, pls. xiv–xv	L; G
16	Holywell, Evershot	Dorset	Warne 1872, 332; Pearce 1983, 471	–
17	Milton Abbas	Dorset	Rowlands 1976, 429	L
18	Tarrant Monkton	Dorset	British Museum registration book for 1892 (9–1.321–5); Rowlands 1976, 233	–
19	Verne Fort	Dorset	Pearce 1983, 429, no. 433	L
20	Whitfield Farm, Beerhacket	Dorset	Arch. J. 1850, 64–5, figs. A–D; Eogan 1967, 145–7	G
21	Circencester	Gloucestershire	Needham 2004, 26–33	M
22	Dundry	Gloucestershire	Adams 2013	M
23	Chalton	Hampshire	Cunliffe 1970	L

2. Combination, composition and context

No.	Location	County	Reference	Code
24	Gable Head, Hayling Island	Hampshire	Rowlands 1976, 239; O'Connor 1980, 321–2, figs. 5–7A	–
25	H.M.S. Sultan, Gosport	Hampshire	Rowlands 1976, 239; O'Connor 1980, 321, fig. 3D	–
26	Liss	Hampshire	Rowlands 1976, 240	L
27	Milton, Portsmouth	Hampshire	Crawford and Wheeler 1921, 139; Rowlands 1976, 242	–
28	South Wonston	Hampshire	Hughes and Champion 1982	–
29	Woolmer Forest	Hampshire	Rowlands 1976, 243–4	–
30	Durley	Hampshire	Hinds 2013	L; G
31	Billingham House?	Hampshire (Isle of Wight)	Rowlands 1976, 240, pl. 17	L
32	Brading Marsh	Hampshire (Isle of Wight)	Roach Smith 1882, 423–4; Rowlands 1976, 238	–
33	Newport	Hampshire (Isle of Wight)	Basford 2012	–
34	Church Farm, Ripple, near Deal	Kent	Parfitt n.d.; B. O'Connor n.d.	–
35	Knight's Bottom Pit, Walmer, Deal	Kent	Parfitt 1994	F
36	St Lawrence's College, Ramsgate	Kent	Hawkes 1942	–
37	Hollicondane, Ramsgate	Kent	Piggott 1949, 118–25	F
38	Langdon Bay, Dover	Kent	Needham et al. 2013, 74–5	L
39	River Medway, Aylesford	Kent	Arch. J. 1873; Roach Smith 1874; Eogan 1994, 128	M
40	South Dumpton Down, Thanet	Kent	Barber 2001, 163	–
41	Unknown, ?Kent	?Kent	Rowlands 1971, 184	L
42	Haxey (Isle of Axholme)	Lincolnshire	Eogan 1967, 149	L
43	Innova Park, Enfield	London	Roberts 2007, 163, no. 108	G
44	'North-east Norfolk'	Norfolk	Varndell 2004, 22–3	–
45	Barton Bendish	Norfolk	Smith 1959a, GB 7, 2 (1–2); Rowlands 1976, 249	L
46	Boughton Fen, Shropham Hundred	Norfolk	Norfolk Museums Service 1977, 27; Lawson 1979	L
47	Bradmoor Common, Pentney	Norfolk	Smith 1959a, 152; Rowlands 1976, 250, pl. 20	G
48	Croxton	Norfolk	Needham 1990, 253–6	–

(Continued on next page)

Appendix 2.1: Middle Bronze Age ornament hoards from Britain (Continued)

No.	Hoard name	County	References	Comment
49	Old Hunstanton	Norfolk	Lawson 1979	–
50	Stoke Ferry	Norfolk	Rowlands 1976, 251; Norfolk Museum Service 1977, 29	–
51	Hopton-on-Sea	Norfolk	Ongoing Treasure case: Treasure report 2012 T73	G
52	Edington Burtle	Somerset	Stradling 1854; Smith 1959b, GB. 44 2(1) & 2(2)	–
53	Monkswood	Somerset	Smith 1959b, GB. 42 2(1) & 2(2)	–
54	Norton Fitzwarren	Somerset	Needham in Ellis 1989, 31–36	M
55	Priddy	Somerset	Payne 2007; Minnitt & Payne 2012	–
56	Spaxton, Quantock Hills	Somerset	Harford 1803, 94, pl., xxiii; Rowlands 1976, 257–8	–
57	Taunton Workhouse	Somerset	Pring 1880; Smith 1959b, GB. 43 2(1) & 2(2)	–
58	Weare	Somerset	Rowlands 1976, 259	–
59	Wedmore	Somerset	Arch. J. 1849, 81; JBAA 1865, 232, pl. 12; Rowlands 1976, 260;	–
60	West Buckland	Somerset	Arch. J. 1880, 107 & plate on opposite page; Taylor 1982	L; M
61	Winterhay Green, Ilminster	Somerset	Evans 1881, 89; Rowlands 1976, 256;	–
62	Lakenheath	Suffolk	Minter 2002	–
63	Thurston	Suffolk	Lawson 1979, 73–5	–
64	Cranleigh	Surrey	Huson 1999	L
65	Falmer Hill, Crawley	Surrey	Holleyman 1948, 60–1; Rowlands 1976, 266	–
66	Ockham	Surrey	Williams 2013	G
67	Binsted ('Binstead' [sic])	Sussex	Varndell 1998/9	L
68	Black Patch, Hut 1	Sussex	Drewett 1982	–
69	Blackrock, Brighton	Sussex	Piggott 1949, 107–31	–
70	Bonchurch Road, Hollingbury	Sussex	PSAL 1901, 409–11; Rowlands 1976, 267–8	–
71	'Brighton/Lewes'	Sussex	Rowlands 1976, 267	F
72	Cowfold	Sussex	Dixon 1849, 268; Rowlands 1976, 266	–
73	East Dean	Sussex	Rowlands 1976, 266	–
74	Hollingbury	Sussex	Arch. J. 1848, 323–5 & plate opposite p. 323	–

75	Jevington	Sussex	British Museum registration book (1991, 0303.1-2)	G
76	Mountfield, Battle	Sussex	Combe 1863, 238–40; Franks 1864; Eogan 1967, 151–2; Taylor 1980, 86	–
77	Newhaven	Sussex	Manley & White 1996	L
78	Pyecombe, Cowdon	Sussex	Rowlands 1976, 268	L
79	South Harting	Sussex	Roberts 2007, 94, no. 91	–
80	Stump Bottom, Cissbury	Sussex	*Antiq. J.* 1926, 444–6; Smith 1959a, 153, fig. 4; Rowlands 1976, 269	–
81	West Ashling	Sussex	S. Needham, British Museum, archive material/notes; Chichester Museum	M
82	'Near Lewes'	Sussex	S. Smith 2011	–
83	Lavant, Chalkpit Lane	Sussex	Kenny 1993	M
84	Durnford	Wiltshire	Annable & Simpson 1964, 621–6	–
85	Elcombe Down, Ebbesbourne Wake	Wiltshire	Rowlands 1976, 271–2	L
86	South Lodge Camp	Wiltshire	Rowlands 1976, 277–8; O'Connor 1991, 234, no. 33	–
87	Scratchbury, Norton Bavant G1	Wiltshire	Colt Hoare 1812, 70; Rowlands 1979, 202, pl. 19	F
88	Wylye	Wiltshire	Ellis 2013	L
89	Cantley	Yorkshire	Needham 2001, 16	–
Wales				
90	Burton, Wrexham	Wales	Gwilt *et al.* 2004	G
91	Capel Isaf	Wales	Savory 1977	L; M
92	Central Wales	Wales	Eogan 1967, 154	G
93	Cwnjenkin Farm, Heyope, Powys	Wales	Savory 1958, 107, 55–6, pl. ii–iv	G
94	Llanwrthwl	Wales	Savory 1958, 52–4, pl. i–ii	G
95	Maesmelan, Powys	Wales	Green *et al.* 1983	L
96	Ogof yr Esgryn Cave, Glyntawe	Wales	Roberts 2007, 165, no. 158	G
97	Tan Llwyn, Clwyd	Wales	Roberts 2007, 165, no. 154	G
98	Tiers Cross, near Milford Haven	Wales	Aldhouse-Green and Northover 1996	L

(Continued on next page)

Appendix 2.1: Middle Bronze Age ornament hoards from Britain (Continued)

No.	Hoard name	County	References	Comment
Scotland				
99	Duff House, Banff, Aberdeenshire	Scotland	Anderson 1883, 446; Coles 1964, 148	G
100	Galloway	Scotland	Wilson 1863, 465; Coles 1964, 147	–
101	Glentrool, Minnigaff, Dumfries & Galloway	Scotland	Callander 1921; Coles 1964, 147	G
102	Lower Largo, Fife	Scotland	Anderson 1884; Eogan 1983, 99, 122	–

Key to comments: F: funerary context; G: goldwork only; M: mixed deposit of copper alloy and goldwork; L: 'less' certain association of objects within the hoard, the remaining hoards are therefore of copper alloy only and of 'more' certain association.

Appendix 2.2: The four most common ornament types and sub-types for hoards of all metal composition types

Ornament type	No. hoards	No. hoards (gold)	No. hoards (gold & copper-alloy)	No. hoards (copper-alloy)
PINS				
Pin: Quoit headed	15	–	1	14
Pin: Decorated	6	–	–	6
Pin: Other types	5	–	1	4
TORCS				
Spiral twisted torc	23		1	22
Flange twisted torc (gold)	19	12	4	15
Ribbon twisted torc	8	6	1	7
Rod torc	1	–	–	1
Cast torc	2	–	–	2
Torc (other types)	3	3	1	2
BRACELET/ARMRING				
B/A Annular (decorated)	13	–	–	13
B/A Annular (undecorated)	11	–	–	11
B/A Penannular (decorated)	7	–	–	7
B/A Penannular (undecorated)	17	8	1	16
Sussex Loops B/A	10		1	9
Spiral twisted B/A	9	1	–	9
Ribbed B/A	7	1	–	7
Double penannular B/A looped ends	2	1	–	2
Ribbon twisted B/A	1		–	1
Twisted wire B/A	1		1	
B/A (other types)	4	3	2	2
'FINGER' RINGS (F/R)				
Spiral F/R	15	1	1	14
Single band F/R	2	1	1	1
Ribbed F/R	6	1	1	5
Composite F/R	1	1	–	1
Ribbon F/R	1		–	1
OTHER				
Rod/wire/tubing	10	3	2	8
Rings	12	2	2	10
Conical 'fittings'	4	–	–	4
Tutuli/domed 'fittings'	3		1	2
Beads	9	1	1	8
Gold sheet objects	2		1	1
Melted objects	1	1	–	1

Key:- B/A: Bracelet/armring; F/R: finger ring.

Chapter 3

Personal objects and personal identity in the Iron Age: the case of the earliest brooches

Sophia Adams

In the mid-fifth century BC a new type of object appeared in Britain: the brooch. From this time on brooches are consistently part of the panoply of metal objects recovered from British sites. From the fifth to second centuries BC they are found in burials, in settlement sites in occupation deposits and pits, and as isolated finds in the landscape. They are small objects that could be clasped to a garment and are shaped in repeated forms although each example is unique and individually crafted. The similarity of form between each brooch, their associations with people through use and deposition, their small personal size and their broad distribution makes them an ideal subject through which to consider and compare their role in dress, personal presentation and, by extension, identity in this period.

The earliest designs share many common traits with examples found on the near continent, yet brooches were in use in Europe for over half a millennium before they appear in Britain (*cf.* Marion 2004; Bietti Sestieri and Macnamara 2007). Although some of these earlier continental brooches are purported to have a British provenance not one has been recovered from a secure archaeological context. The evidence instead indicates these arrived in Britain after the Iron Age and many appear to be antiquarian imports given artificial British provenances (Hull and Hawkes 1987, 7–8; Adams 2013, 101–3). Approximately 720 brooches are known in England, Scotland and Wales from *c.* 450–150 BC, the Early and Middle Iron Age (Adams 2013). After this time the quantity increases dramatically with more than 15,000 brooches dating to the last century BC (Mackreth 2011). Previous research on the social and personal significance of brooches in Britain has focussed on the Late Iron Age (post-150 BC) (e.g. Fox 1927; Alexander 1973; Hill 1995; Hattatt 1982; 1985; 1987; 1989; Haselgrove 1997; Jundi and Hill 1998; Eckardt 2008; Mackreth 2011). This is in part owing to the increased quantity of finds relating to personal dress and adornment during that period. Sophia Jundi and J. D. Hill saw this as a significant shift in emphasis on personal appearance they equated with an 'emergence of the individual' (Jundi and Hill 1998, 129–30). Hella Eckardt has criticised this as an over-simplified analysis and instead equates the increased quantity of such artefacts with a more vague indication of a time of changes in the modes by which people 'presented themselves to others' (Eckardt 2008, 114). This chapter addresses the earlier evidence to question whether brooches can provide clues to the changing ways in which people presented themselves to others, which in turn might lead to insights about the idea of the individual. I will examine the Early and Middle Iron Age brooches in Britain from *c.* 450-150 BC particularly from burials but also non-burial contexts to ascertain what they were attached to, in what position and where on the body they were found, and how they might have been worn and viewed. By discussing this contextual evidence we may explore their significance in terms of personal identity and appearance. This will demonstrate the value of Early and Middle Iron Age brooches in the study of dress and identity in Iron Age Britain. The focus rests primarily on brooches to address existing interpretations of the role of these objects and to provide a starting point for future comparisons across the entire Iron Age period which could incorporate other dress associated objects that have been excluded from this chapter owing to the demands of space.

Early and Middle Iron Age brooches

The earliest form of brooch found and manufactured in Britain is the bronze bow brooch. This consists of a pin to pierce the fabric, a convex, flat or concave bow parallel to the pin, a spring or hinge (at the head of the brooch) to create tension between the bow and pin enabling the brooch to be opened, and a catchplate (at the foot of the brooch) in which to insert the pin to hold the brooch shut (Fig. 3.1). On Early Iron Age examples (*c.* 450-300 BC) the foot is usually reverted (bent back towards the bow) (Types 1A and 1B, Fig. 3.2) (Hull and Hawkes 1987, 72; Adams 2013, 52). The first brooches to appear in Britain are the Type 1A stylistically, which are contemporary with the fifth century BC type (La Tène I or La Tène A) found on the Continent and often referred to as Marzabotto brooches (Smith 1905; Fox 1923; Hodson 1964; Hull and Hawkes 1987; Marion 2004). These have a high arched bow and large coiled springs (Figs. 3.1 and 3.2, Type 1A). Despite the similar overall shape to their Continental counterparts the British examples are often smaller and more simply decorated implying they are locally manufactured versions of the form. Early Iron Age brooches range in size from 25mm to 76mm and are typically made of bronze (less than 3% are iron). Middle Iron Age brooches are as common in iron as bronze (Adams 2013, 174) and the latter tend to be particularly small, *c.* 30mm long. From *c.* 375 BC the British brooches show greater variation in structural form and have simpler decoration than their European counterparts, these are classified as the 1B brooches found in England and Wales (Fig. 3.2 nos. 2–4).

In the Middle Iron Age (*c.* 300–150 BC) the end of the reverted foot of the brooch is either wrapped around the bow or attached to it with a separate collar (Type 2A and 2C,

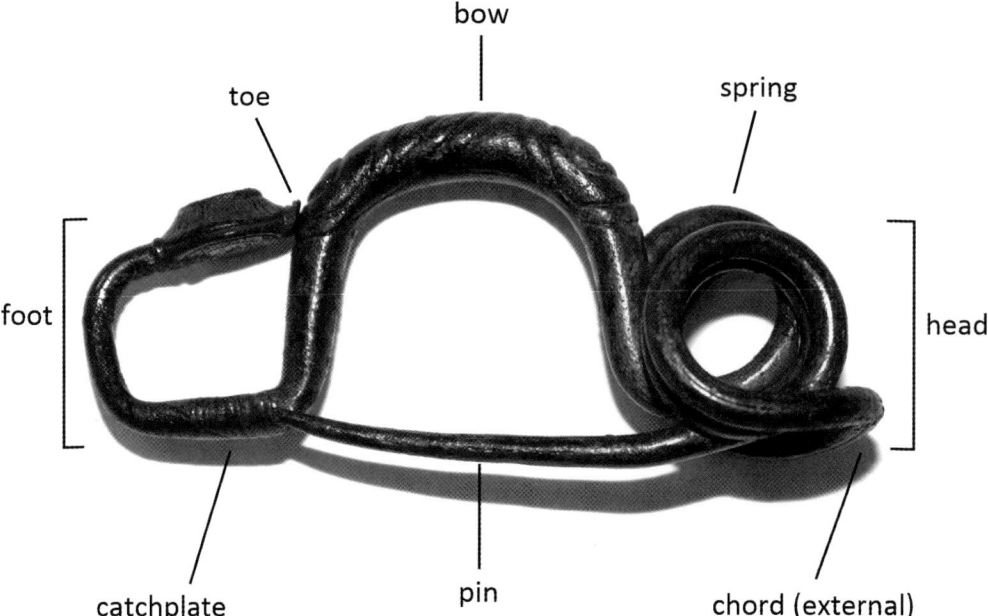

Fig. 3.1: Parts of an Iron Age bow brooch. (Adams 2013, 22 fig. 2). Early Iron Age Type 1A brooch. Box, Wiltshire (BM 1906, 1113.1) (photograph by S. Adams ©Trustees of the British Museum).

Fig. 3.2). Occasionally the bow, catchplate and foot are cast as a single solid piece (See Type 2L, Fig. 3.2, nos. 14 and 15). British brooches become even more distinctive from Continental ones at this time. Insular types, that is those particular to Britain, include the concave bowed involuted brooches (Type 2C, Fig. 3.2, Adams 2013, 59). Despite the chronological connections in the style of foot the earlier foot forms do continue into later phases so this feature alone cannot be a precise chronological indicator.

During the Middle Iron Age (*c.* 300-150 BC) plate brooches appear alongside the bow brooches (Type 2B, Fig. 3.2). These become even more common in later periods. The earliest plate forms consist of an upper surface that is visible when attached to cloth. This is the shaped, decorative part or plate. It hides the hinged pin mechanism attached to the back of the brooch. They tend to be of moulded bulbous shapes or inlaid with other materials such as coral (Adams 2013, 64–8).

Early and Middle Iron Age brooches have been found in burials (136 brooches at 23 sites) in settlements (74 brooches at 44 sites), at hillforts (94 brooches at 32 sites), in watery locations, typically riverine inter-tidal zones (35 brooches from 12 sites), at dryland ritualised contexts disassociated from settlement or subsistence activity (93 brooches from 9 sites) and occasionally on Late Iron Age and Roman period sites (14 brooches from 11 sites) (Adams 2013, 186, see Figs. 3.3 and 3.4). Over 240 brooches of definite Early Iron Age type have been recorded but less than 50 were found during archaeological excavation. The majority were recovered from scattered find-spots often by metal detecting activity and reported to the Portable Antiquities

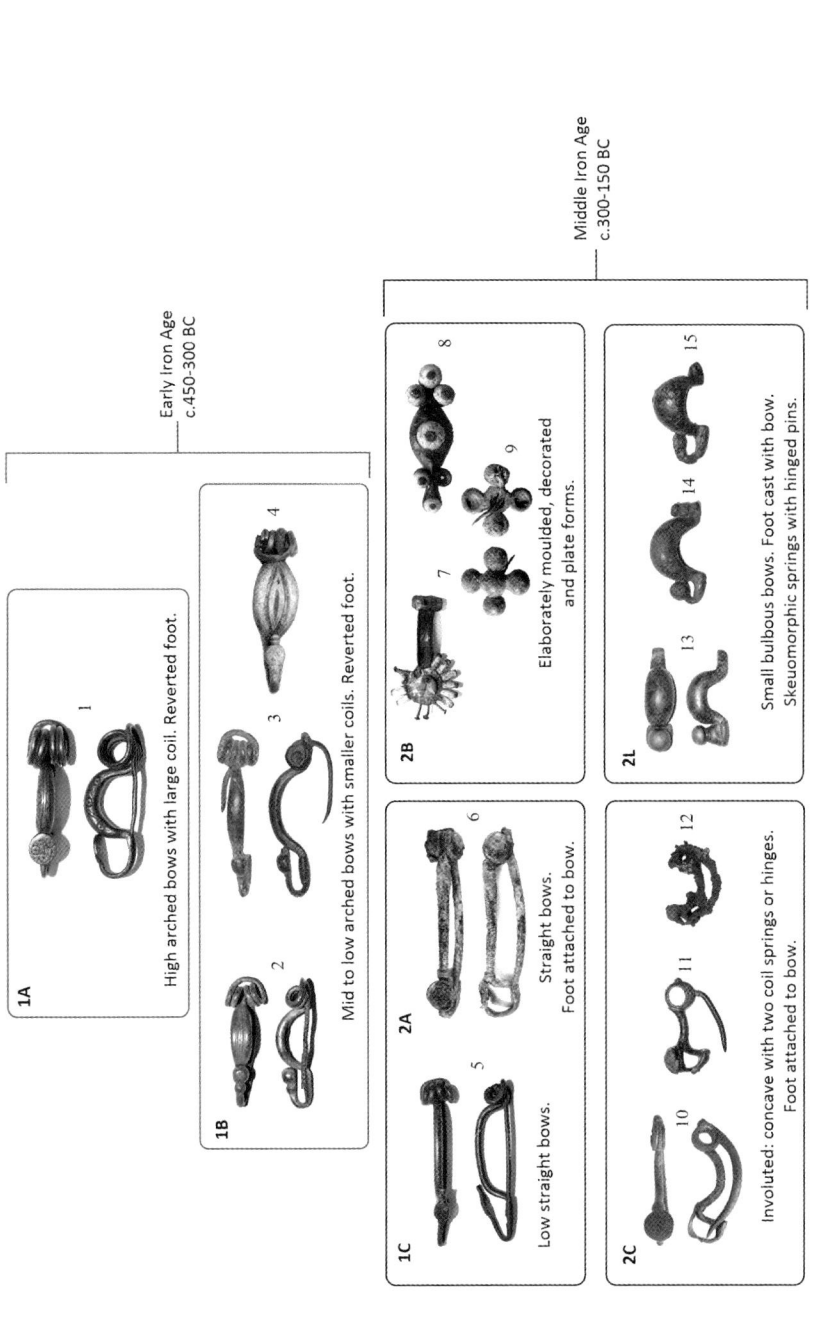

Fig. 3.2: Simple typology of Early and Middle Iron Age brooches. (after Adams 2015, fig. 3). 1: Middle Hill, Woodeaton, Oxfordshire (BM 1880,1214.13); 2: Bryanston Farm, Blandford, Dorset (1892,0901.1572); 3: Dorset (PAS: DOR-41F0C6); 4: Greater London (PAS: SUR-0B2C37); 5: Abingdon, Oxon (BM 1904,1213.1); 6: Argam Lane, Rudston, East Riding of Yorks (BM 1978,1202.14); 7: Harborough Cave, Brassington, Derbys (BM 1951,1102.1); 8: Mill Hill, Deal (BM 1990,0102.25); 9: Berkhire (PAS: BERK-4EFFC6); 10: W. Yorks. (PAS: SWYOR-399938); 11: Makeshift Cemetery, East Riding of Yorks (BM1975,0401.36); 12: Bell Slack, East Riding of Yorks (BM 1978,1203.7); 13: Hammersmith, London (BM 1898,0618.27); 14: Surrey (PAS: SUR-41D522); 15: Snodland, Kent (BM 1993,0501.1) (BM finds) (PAS finds reproduced under Creative Commons Share-Alike Agreement). Photographs S. Adams ©Trustees of the British Museum;

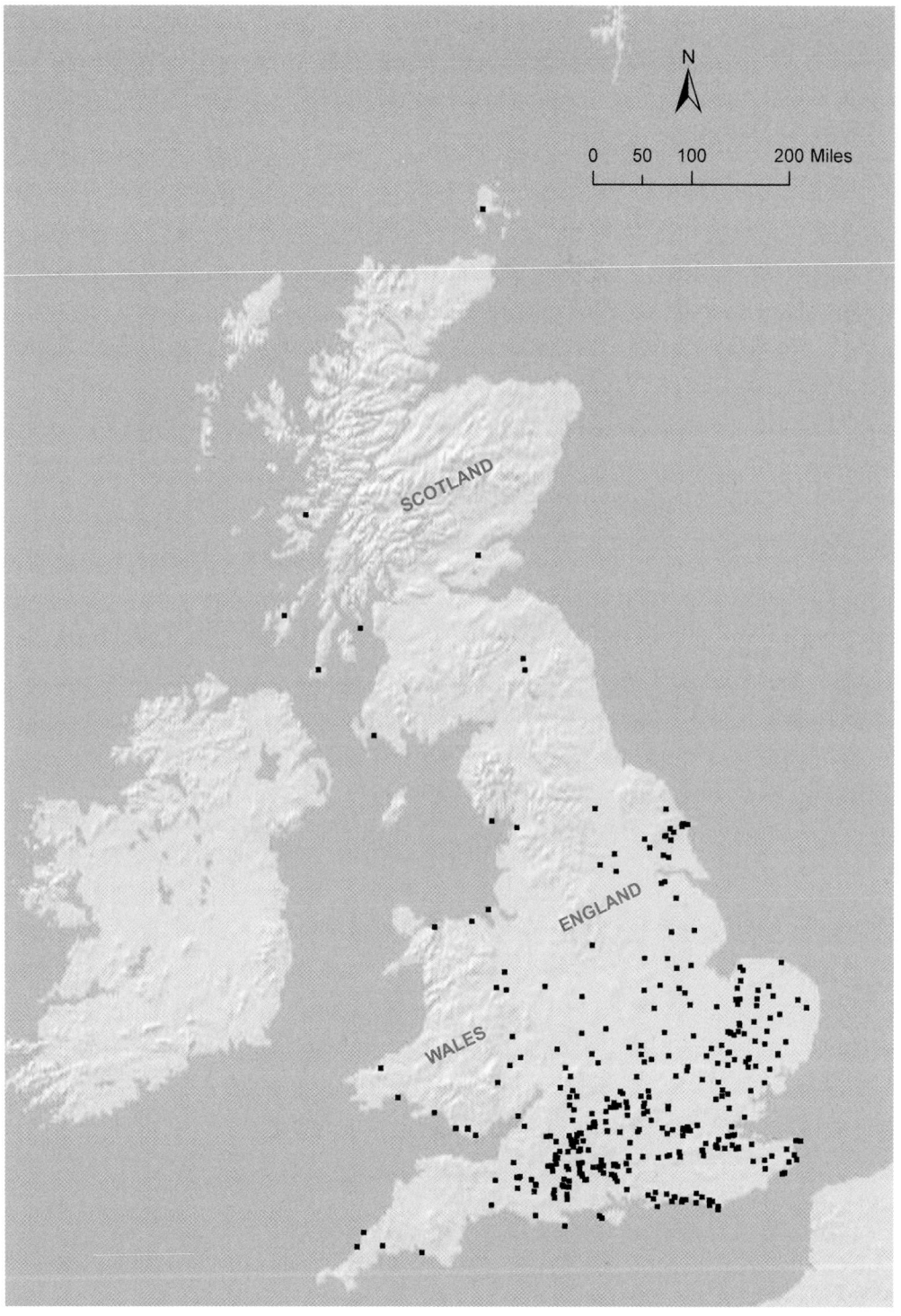

Fig. 3.3: Distribution of findspots of Early and Middle Iron Age brooches in Britain (after Adams 2014, 175, fig. 2).

3. Personal objects and personal identity in the Iron Age

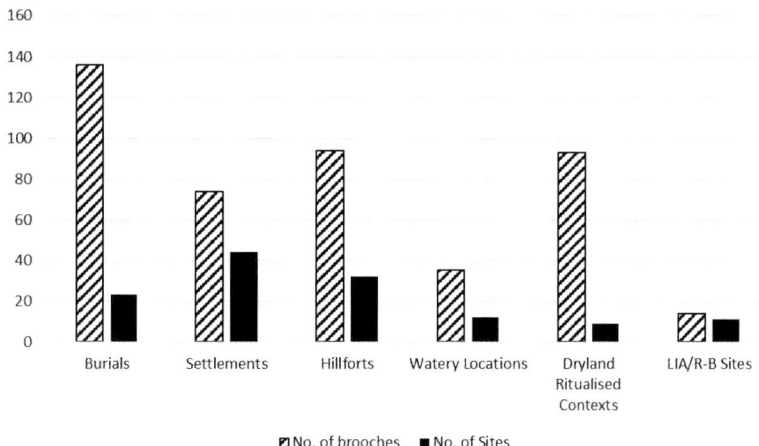

Fig. 3.4: Overview of the context of Early and Middle Iron Age brooches, including excavated and stray finds from known sites (data from Adams 2013, 181-4). The Thames has been treated as four findspots: the City, East London, West London and upstream west of London.

Scheme (Adams 2013, 169), a number of these have landscape type or subsequent archaeological site associations. Greater numbers of Middle Iron Age brooches are found than in the preceding period and the majority of these (240 out of 300 brooches) have been recovered from excavations. The remainder of the brooches are in too fragmentary a state to assign to a specific Early or Middle Iron Age type.

The greatest quantities of brooches from any type of feature are those from burials: 135 were found in graves in cemeteries and one with a burial in a pit within the settlement at Slonk Hill, West Sussex (Hartridge 1978, 80). Four of the brooches in burials are of Early Iron Age type the remainder are Middle Iron Age. The burial evidence is vital to our understanding of the relationship between brooches, dress and the body. It provides the closest direct association of brooches with the human body and clothing for a time when we lack contemporary written descriptions and illustrations depicting people in Britain. Even then we must be cautious in equating the burial evidence, the fabric and accoutrements from graves, with the dress of the living, as discussed below.

Most Early and Middle Iron Age brooches entered the archaeological record separate from people. In Middle Iron Age settlements the features in which brooches are found are usually pits but at hillforts there is very little evidence for structured deposition of brooches in features. Revised Early and Middle Iron Age data show these brooches are also rare finds in boundary features (Adams 2013, 224–5) contra to results achieved almost two decades ago (Haselgrove 1997, 55). In fact brooches are most frequently recovered from general occupation layers: layers of material that have built up during settlement activity rather than being specifically laid down in a feature (Adams 2013, 224–5). In these cases there is a physical separation of the brooch from the individual. A similar situation can be seen at the ritualised dryland site at

Grandcourt Farm, Middleton, Norfolk. Here 38 Middle Iron Age bronze brooches were found in an amorphous spread of material overlying a line of pits, containing complete pottery vessels, cut into a natural gulley down the side of a natural promontory (Adams *et al.* forthcoming). Similarities in the style and decoration of the brooches suggest they are all roughly contemporary.

Social identities and brooches

As visually complex objects, brooches could have been encoded with meaning not only in their form and decoration but also the materials from which they were made and how they were worn (Wells 2008, 40–1). Alfred Gell warns us that objects and their decoration cannot be read like texts because they are not structured like language (Gell 1998, 163–5). It is the physical properties of the object, its tactile qualities and location within the context of other Iron Age objects that formed the basis from which the object was understood. Anthropological research on clothing has explored the complex relationship between dress and personal identity (e.g. Miller 2010). Daniel Miller's comparison of clothing and attitudes to dress in Trinidad, India and London highlights not only the culturally specific nature of how clothes are perceived to represent the wearer but also how peoples' feelings about themselves are affected through cultural attitudes towards dress and personal interaction with clothing (Miller 2010, 23–38). Garments may be worn to present a certain idea of oneself and/or by wearing certain styles of garment in certain ways one may feel a certain way or adopt character traits. Yet as Joanna Brück has warned we should not imagine that all individuals in the past or present are free to act as they wish, such freedom of the individual is a European cultural construct since the eighteenth century (Brück 2006, 74–5). This is not to say that we cannot examine the question of personal identity in the Iron Age but we must be aware that an individual's choice may have been controlled, restricted and manipulated by persons other than themselves, or by a group as a whole. A person may not have been seen to act alone, their actions always affecting and being affected by the group. Brooches as a part of Iron Age dress and as items connected to personal appearance are tied into these complex issues of personal presentation and representation. To contemplate the possible role of brooches in presenting, influencing or manipulating personal or group identity at this time we need to examine the evidence for people's interaction with these objects through the specific contexts in which they are found and their physical qualities.

Brooches in burials

A general shift is visible during the Iron Age from brooches being exceptionally rare items in burials at the start of the period in the Early Iron Age (see above), to being relatively common at the end, in the Late Iron Age (e.g. Fitzpatrick 1997; Mackreth 2011).

However the pattern is not consistent across Britain hinting at the precedence of regional preferences. Middle Iron Age brooches have been found in burials in England only, typically in the same regions which have evidence for a cemetery style funerary rite: in the East Riding of Yorkshire, Cornwall, Hampshire, Kent, Cambridgeshire, and Lincolnshire (Fig. 3.5). The exception being the aforementioned burial in a pit at Slonk Hill, Sussex (Hartridge 1978, 80). The evidence is concentrated on the Middle Iron Age cemeteries of the Yorkshire Wolds (East Riding of Yorkshire) but even here the brooch evidence is still limited. Of the 446 burials at the Wetwang Slack cemetery, only 41 contained bow brooches (Dent 1982, 437, 442). At Mill Hill, Deal, Kent the percentage of graves containing brooches was also close to 10% but this accounts for only four out of 42 burials. In other cemeteries the numbers are even lower with only one or two burials containing Middle Iron Age brooches such as the single grave with a brooch in the cemetery at Suddern Farm, Hampshire (Cunliffe and Poole 2000, 168) or Harlyn Bay in Cornwall where out of 130 graves only two contained brooches (Hull and Hawkes 1987, 52). We must remain cautious when extrapolating these modes of dress to the wider population especially considering the extremely small sample of the population that were buried in the ground and the even lower frequency of brooches in these graves. The small numbers of brooches in burials across England at this time, especially in comparison to contemporary Continental cemeteries (e.g. Bretz Mahler 1971; Stead and Rigby 1999; Evans 2004; Desenne et al. 2009), may be just as indicative of differences in burial practices as of different attitudes to these objects or different modes of dress. As a result we cannot know for sure that the Suddern Farm brooch, for instance, is an anomaly or a significant adornment for the individual with whom it was buried but both the fact that this woman was buried in this way and with a brooch may be significant.

Iron brooches are more prevalent in burials than bronze brooches whereas the latter are more common in watery locations and dryland sites of a ritualised character. This could indicate differential selection for each deposition practice or even that iron brooches were designed more to be worn than placed in ritually significant locations. The latter argument is not supported by the higher frequency of bronze brooches as single finds in the landscape nor does it take into consideration the higher probability that heavily corroded iron brooches are recovered from carefully excavated graves contexts compared to watery environments and metal-detected plough soil. The choice of metal appears to reflect regional practices: the majority of burials containing brooches are in the Yorkshire Wolds in relatively close proximity to natural iron ore sources in particular the iron production centre of the Foulness Valley (Halkon 2008). In contrast most of the brooches found in watery contexts are derived from the Thames and other southern waterways at some distance from the sources of copper and tin in western England, Wales and across the Channel. Bronze brooches also appear to be preferred for deposition at sites set apart from settlement activity, without human burials but with organised, ritualised, deposition of specific complete artefacts such as Grandcourt Farm, Middleton, Norfolk. These sites are also

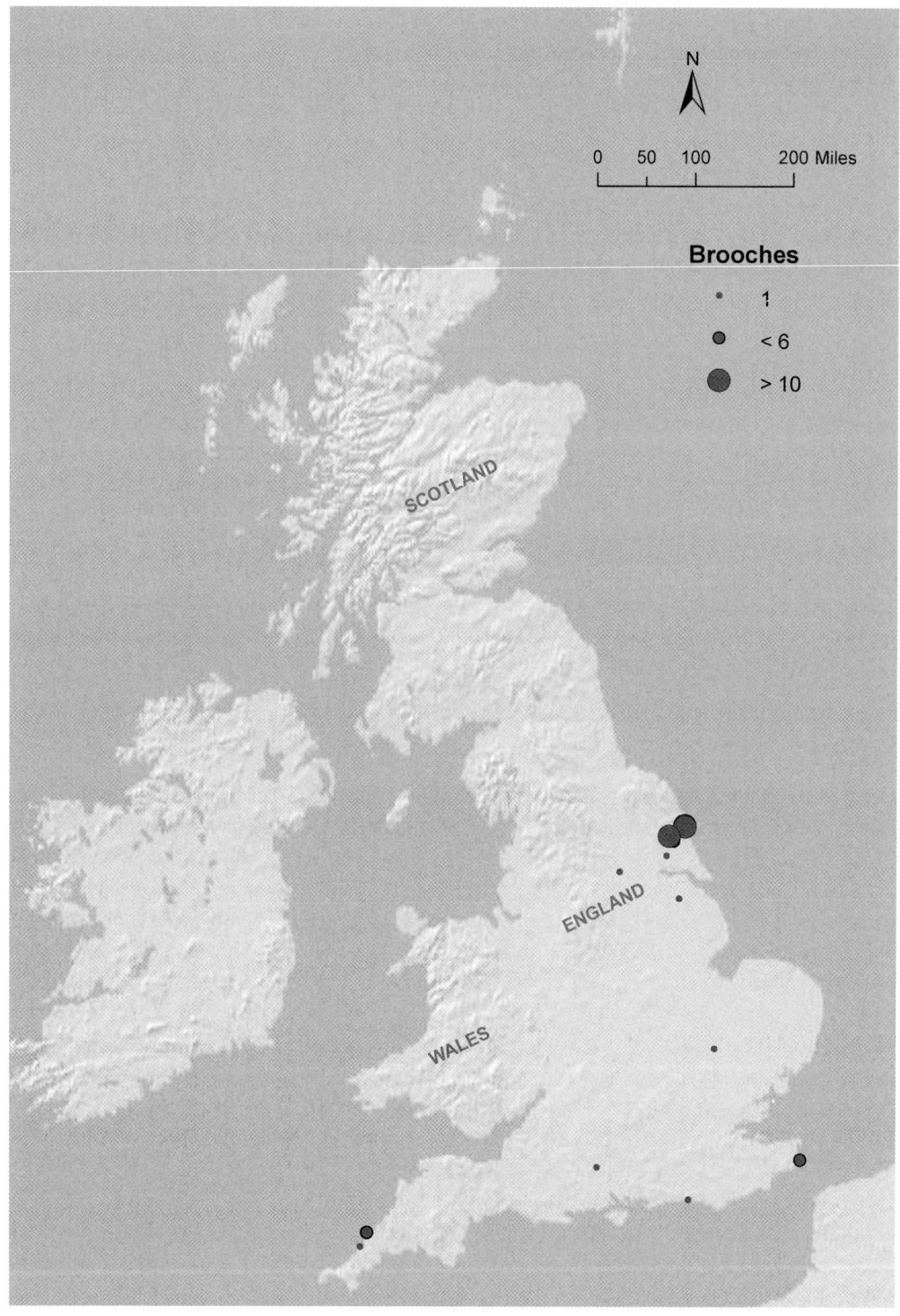

Fig. 3.5: Location and quantity of brooches found in burials (after Adams 2013, 268 map 7.7).

located in areas where contemporary brooches are not found in burials (Figs. 3.3 and 3.5). Beyond Yorkshire, bronze brooches are almost as common in burials as iron brooches (eight bronze to nine iron). The people of the Yorkshire Wolds were making use of locally available and locally significant materials. Certainly the choice of material for the brooches appears to be tied up with regional ritual deposition practices as well as the local importance of different metals (Adams 2014) but the value may also have been placed on more distantly transported metals. Perhaps it is significant that ritually deposited brooches were of these non-local materials while in the Yorkshire Wolds the connection between local people and the value of their local resources was highlighted in the brooches in the burials. But, this does not account for the rarity of bronze brooches here or their more frequent presence in burials elsewhere in England.

No simple equation can be drawn between the relative richness of the grave and the inclusion of a brooch of a particular metal. But it is interesting to note that brooches decorated with additional materials, such as opaque glass (Fig. 3.2 nos. 6 and 11) or coral (Fig. 3.2 nos. 7 and 8), are more commonly found in burials than any other context. Just over half of the 80 brooches decorated in this manner have been found in burial contexts (Adams 2013, 229). Glass inlaid examples are only found in burials, and of the 24 coral-inlaid brooches 64% were found in graves. Of the eight coral-inlaid brooches in non-burial contexts, two were found in specific features relating to ramparts: one at Castle Yard, Farthingstone in a deposit of collapsed rampart material (Knight 1987, 26–7), and the other was disturbed from the rampart bank at Maiden Castle, Dorset (Wheeler 1943, 257). A further example was recovered from Harborough Cave, Derbyshire (Fig. 3.2 no. 7) (Smith 1909) along with a variety of artefacts suggesting repeated deposition of important objects that could be viewed as votive or certainly indicative of rituals that required the transfer of objects up to and into the cave. Although taphonomic processes could account for the lack of coral on non-burial brooches, the lack of suitable brooch forms in those contexts implies there is a preference towards depositing brooches decorated with extra materials in graves as opposed to in any other features or environments (Adams 2013, 229). Two further brooches found in non-funerary contexts at Flag Fen, Cambridgeshire and Meare Lake Village, Somerset were probably once decorated with coral but that material is now missing; Dent (1995) has proposed that it was deliberately removed prior to deposition. Coral was a rare material at this time, perhaps imported from the Mediterranean or collected as rare stems washed up on the North Sea coast (Adams 2013, 158–9). Coral's rarity on Iron Age objects in general and its absence on Late Iron Age artefacts, indicates that access to this material was limited. The possibility that it was removed from some artefacts to decorate others only increases the perception of its rarity and by extension its high value. On the Continent, evidence for the restriction to the supply of coral but continued desire for it may be observed in the recycling of smaller and smaller pieces during the period and the use of substitutes to produce the appearance of coral (Champion 1982, 68; Fürst 2010, 138). The evidence is not conclusive but it is suggestive that the display qualities of the brooches were important for those included in funerary garb.

Dressing the dead or the dress of the living

Where corroded brooches are found in graves they are always fused in a shut position showing they probably entered the grave clasped to cloth or were removed and closed prior to deposition. Support for the former may be found in the presence of mineralised fibres or casts of fibres in corrosion deposits on some iron brooches. For example, a woollen cloak border from grave BF20 Burton Fleming, East Riding of Yorkshire was preserved in the corrosion from a small iron brooch (Stead 1991, 214; Crowfoot 1991, 119–21). Altogether cloth remains were found on only *c.* 10% of the inhumed bodies in the Yorkshire Wold cemeteries (Dent 1982, 437, 442) but the presence of brooches on top of or close to the skeletal remains suggests far more graves contained human remains buried in clothing or wrapped in fabric. There appears to be no single set place on the body where the brooch was located; they are found at the shoulder or chest, in front of the face, on top of the legs, beside the neck, against an elbow or at the waist. This variety has previously been identified in Yorkshire Wold graves (Giles 2012, 130), but is also true for examples from the rest of England. On the burial of a man on a wheeled vehicle at Ferry Fryston, West Yorkshire, and the burial of a woman in a pit at Slonk Hill, West Sussex, the brooches are located at the shoulders of both skeletons. A brooch was found in the waist area of the extended inhumation at Bromfield, Shropshire (Hughes 1994), and on a flexed burial at Suddern Farm, Hampshire (Cunliffe and Poole 2000). Although the bones are poorly preserved at Trethellan Farm, Newquay, Cornwall (Nowakowski 1991), the surviving remains and position within the grave cuts show the brooches were found at the heads of two individuals. Single brooches were located at the elbows of two skeletons at Mill Hill Deal, Kent (graves 108 and 127) and at the chest in another (grave 47). Many of these positions would be impractical for everyday wear: a brooch at the shoulder could have remained comfortably attached during activity or at the waist if on a tunic, but a brooch at the elbow would restrict movement, one in front of the face would hinder vision and on the legs could limit the gait. We are reliant on the accuracy of the excavation and recording process for asserting such claims about brooch positioning, as we are for all our analysis of excavated data. Although it is possible that excavation processes could have shifted the position of the brooch before recording, the methods for excavating skeletal remains mean it is unlikely to have affected the relative position of the human remains and artefacts in these cases.

To explain these various brooch positions we may compare those burials with brooches to those containing no durable artefacts (Giles 2012, 131). In the Yorkshire Wolds, Giles noted that 66% of the burials fall into the latter category and many of these bodies appear to have been placed in wooden coffins, whereas the former group with artefacts appear not to have been placed in coffins (*ibid.*). The coffin would have encased the body covering it and making it easier to lift the deceased into the grave. For the non-coffin burials the bodies may instead have been bound and covered by fabric forming a shroud. The fabric could have been wound around the body and the loose end secured with a brooch, pin, or even an organic toggle or tie. The position of each brooch might indicate merely the location at which the loose end of the cloth was secured. If this were the case then the varied positions of the brooches shows that there was no set route for winding the cloth around the body or different lengths of fabric were used thereby reaching different points at the end of the wrapping. The corrosion deposits have shown this fabric to be a thorn-proof, water-resistant woollen material suited to use as a cloak (Crowfoot 1991, 119). It is not unfeasible then to imagine the shroud was formed by wrapping a cloak around the flexed body, perhaps the deceased's own cloak (Bretz-Mahler 1971; Giles 2012, 130). In extended inhumations where the brooch tends to be located down the central axis of the body or at the chest then the cloak may simply have been folded round the body in the manner in which it was worn in life.

The function of brooches in the head area can perhaps be explained as clasps on a shroud covering the face of the deceased (Giles 2012, 130). Once wrapped in this way the deceased would be recognisable only from their bodily form and material possessions (Adams 2013, 219). If the shrouds were formed from an outer garment such as cloak it may be that cloaks were both items of cover (in life and death) and personal display. Mineralised fibres from Burton Fleming and Rudston burials show the presence of different weaves and dyed yarns that would have produced patterns in the fabric (Crowfoot 1991, 119–21). The cloak with its fine weave, stripes, colours and decorated borders would be a key item of display for an Iron Age person. A brightly shining brooch could have been just one part of this visual panoply rather than necessarily the centrepiece. The manufacturing processes of lost wax casting and forging (Adams 2013, 140–61) meant that each brooch was unique even if similar in form to other examples. The specific colours and decoration on each cloak and the brooch used to pin it may be directly associated with the deceased individual. Alternatively these possessions could have been bestowed on the dead by another, thereby visibly connecting a living individual with the deceased. If the woollen cloth was woven specifically for wrapping the dead body this brings up the question of whether such cloth was woven in preparation for the inevitable death of someone in the social group or was specifically made for the individual who was buried wrapped up in it. In the latter case we face the issue of the time it takes to produce such a cloth. The bodies buried in this fabric are articulated and the skeletons show neither signs of exposure burial nor a long period of time between death and deposition. Assuming time would not have been available to make a new woollen wrapping between death and burial then it is possible such fabric was stored during life in preparation for an individual's inevitable demise. This leads us back to the possibility that if a woollen outer garment, big enough to wrap around a person, was used in life it could feasibly be used to wrap the person when they died thereby retaining the personal connection between cloth, body and personal identity. These subtle differences could have connected each object with the individual wearer.

Middle Iron Age brooches always appear to be located in a position where it would be visible when the deceased was laid in the grave, whether in an extended or crouched inhumation, whether in a long grave cut or a reused pit. None have been found underneath the human remains (Adams 2013, 219–21). This emphasises the importance of the visual effect of a brooch in the funerary process. At Mill Hill Deal, in Grave 112 the coral-decorated brooch (Fig. 3.2 no. 8) was found face down over the deceased's left tibia (Parfitt 1995, 18). This does not necessarily mean it was laid in the grave thus; in fact the position may be the result of it falling as the organic material to which it was attached decomposed. For this grave it has been proposed that the brooch was attached to fabric (perhaps a cloak) folded and placed on top of the shins (*ibid*.). The positioning of the body and the objects in this grave implies the importance of viewing the deceased wearing fine bronze ornaments and with a sword and shield at his sides and perhaps his cloak resting on his legs. They did not want to enshroud the deceased but it was still important to include the cloak in the grave. If viewing was important the grave must have been left open for a period of time after the body was laid in it, perhaps only for a day or a fire-lit night but at least providing enough time for the relevant people to see the furnished grave. Viewing in this case would be part of the funerary ritual and may have been passive or more interactive such as the placing of animal remains or artefacts in the grave with the deceased as in the case of the Wetwang Village chariot burial (Hill 2001). Possible examples of graves left open for viewing range from Cornwall to Kent to Yorkshire.

People and their brooches

Brooches are found in burials of both male and female adults aged from *c*. 17 to 50+ (Hartridge 1978, 80; Parfitt 1995, 159–70; Cunliffe and Poole 2000, 168; Giles 2012, 132). No brooches have been found buried with children in Britain. Iron Age child burials are scarce but it is of note that brooches are also absent from children's graves on the Continent with the exception of the Bucy-le-Long cemetery in Aisne, France where the Dux type of brooch was found exclusively in children's graves (Desenne *et al*. 2009, 445). It seems that for the majority of Iron Age children a brooch was not part of their dress. As Joanna Sofaer Derevenski has argued: the presence of certain artefacts and the physical association of the child's skeletal remains with the grave may 'be regarded as the material manifestation of the interaction between child and society' (Sofaer Derevenski 2000, 10). The fact that brooches, and other metal artefact types, are recovered from some adult graves but are absent from children's graves is a part of this social interaction. It does not enable us to reconstruct exactly the contemporary concept of child but it does indicate a differentiation was made between juveniles and biological mature adults in the funerary realm that must have been influenced by attitudes to living children. The biological age association of brooches could reflect attitudes towards either the giving of these rare items to adults as opposed to children or it could be part of a conscious choice not to include these objects in the rare cases when a child was buried in a manner that is archaeologically visible. This does not necessarily mean that children did not wear brooches, but such objects could have been passed on to those who eventually reached maturity. Giles has noted that greater quantities of durable objects or 'belongings' are found in adult as opposed to juvenile burials in the Yorkshire Wold graves (Giles 2012, 132). In fact the percentage of graves containing such objects increases with the age of the deceased up to a maximum of 50% for all the oldest adult graves aged 45+ years (*ibid.*). In the Yorkshire Wolds at least, material objects, particularly those associated with personal adornment do appear to be connected with age. They could relate to the veneration of an older person upon their death or these unique objects may have been accumulated during a person's life.

Roughly equal numbers of brooches are found in adult male and female graves in East Yorkshire (Stead 1991, 90). Despite the low frequency of Iron Age burials elsewhere in Britain and the even lower occurrence of brooches in these graves, where they do occur there is still no definitive bias towards burial with men or women. In southern England in the Middle Iron Age cemetery at Mill Hill, Deal, three males were buried with brooches and only one female (Parfitt 1995, 159–70). In Hampshire the only example is a female burial in the cemetery at Suddern Farm (Cunliffe and Poole 2000, 168). At Slonk Hill, West Sussex, of the two burials on the site one was male without a brooch and one female with a brooch (Hartridge 1978, 80). Brooches of the same shape and material are found in both adult female and male graves. Where the bodies can be independently sexed there is also no visible bias in the positioning of brooches in any grave nor does there appear to be a meaningful distinction between the size of brooches worn by men and women. John Dent proposed that the smaller brooches were more frequently associated with women in the Yorkshire Wold cemeteries (Dent 1982, 443, fig. 5) but this is the result of the manner in which he has divided different types rather than a true reflection of the gendered associations which actually show that longer brooches occur with women or men in different cemeteries or have no bias at all (Adams 2013, 218). Brooches are found in burials with blue beads that have been positively connected to older women (Fitzpatrick 2007, 345; Giles 2008, 72) but they also occasionally occur with shields (Ferry Fryston and Mill Hill Deal) and swords (Mill Hill Deal) that have been shown to have a direct connection with biological males in a burial context (Stead 1991, 33). Brooches have also been found with adult males of about 25–35 years old with evidence for possible injuries incurred through fighting. (Stead 1991, 185–211; Giles 2008, 66). A brooch could be part of a well-furnished male or female grave or it could be the only inorganic object in a grave. It might be used to clasp the shroud round an injured man's corpse or it might hold the wrapping around the only woman buried in a single settlement, as at Slonk Hill (Hartridge 1978, 80).

Brooches do not appear to be an explicit part of the construction of gender identity in England in the Middle Iron Age if such identity was intertwined with biological sex as recognised in the skeletal remains (Whitehouse 2007, 31; Sørensen 2007, 46). They could be an indicator of equality between men and women, where social difference is not specifically marked by being either a woman or a man. We find examples of richly furnished graves of both women and men from the Middle Iron Age and a few of these also contain the less common coral decorated brooches such as that buried with a man in the aforementioned Mill Hill Grave 112. An iron brooch was found amongst the beaded cord tie of a pelt bag covering an iron mirror in the female chariot burial at Wetwang Village, it was thought to have been attached to this cord (Hill 2001; Joy 2010). The latter case demonstrates that occasionally brooches might also be attached to accessories, in this case associated with a potent and rare object: the mirror (Joy 2010, 79; 2011). The complex associations of different objects and biological sex may well be the result of the complexity of gender identity in the Middle Iron Age. The oft-cited examples of the Sambia and Hua Papua New Guinea (Herdt 1987; e.g. Parker Pearson 1999, 101; Whitehouse 2007, 32–5) reminds us that an individual's gender may be understood to alter over time through cultural intervention or natural processes or a combination of both without these being considered to be different forces at work. The lack of patterning of brooch evidence in adult graves makes it difficult to ascertain their specific relationship to possible developmental or changing stages in people's lives and prompts us to wonder if their relevance to the individual has a bearing beyond life cycles punctuated by physical and biological change.

Wearing a brooch

Many brooches from c. 450-150 BC are too small to grasp a large amount of fabric, especially a thick fabric, for example the tiny 25mm long 2L brooches (Fig. 3.2 nos. 13–15) and the majority of bronze Type 2C brooches. They also have only shallow catchplates that would have acted more as a rest for the pin than a secure holder. These small brooches certainly appear to be better suited to adorning fabric rather than holding swathes of fabric or clasping a garment in place. Given the generally small dimensions of the British brooches, one might also think they had a less dramatic effect on the viewer than the Continental forms, but these small shiny objects would have been easily distinguished against the background of a cloak. Light reflected from a polished golden looking bronze or silvery iron brooch would have drawn attention to this item when attached to more light absorbent materials such as woven wool. For many graves the brooch is the only shiny metallic item in the burial, although they are also found in more abundantly furnished burials such as the burials with wheeled vehicles at Wetwang Village burial, East Riding of Yorkshire, (Hill 2001; Joy 2010) and Ferry Fryston burial in West Yorkshire (Brown et al. 2007, 147). It was not necessary to use a large brooch to achieve this vibrant effect. The glint may have drawn the viewer in to gain a better look at the brooch. At close range the shape and decorative detail on the brooch becomes visible. The glint and the curved shape indicated the presence of a brooch, which acted as a badge for the viewer to ponder.

The majority of Early and Middle Iron Age bow brooches had an omnidirectional form in that the shape could be enjoyed from the side or from above and with the brooch positioned at any angle. The designs do not appear to be aimed at only one viewing plane. The correct way of wearing a brooch was therefore in a visible location on the front of the body or outside of a bag but the designs do not show us which way up was preferred or acceptable. It is possible that meaning lay in the orientation of the brooch but we can only speculate on this possibility. In other examples we see hints that the meaning lay within the form of the visible part of the brooch. For example, the bulbous cruciform 2B brooch (Fig. 3.2 no. 9) would have been indistinguishable from pins with a similar shaped head, such those found at Fairfield Park, Stotfold, Bedfordshire and Ludford, Lincolnshire (Allen and Webley 2007, 94), when attached to fabric. Only the mechanism by which they were attached to the fabric would distinguish one object type (the brooch) from the other (the pin). The case of the similar pins and brooches hints at the possibility that for these specific objects the final visual effect was the intended outcome and not the manner in which this was achieved. This is further supported by the assemblage of 38 bronze brooches found at Grandcourt Farm, Norfolk (Adams *et al.* forthcoming). Ten different spring and hinge forms are used but these produce only four different shapes of brooch: in other words the same overall shape is achieved using different construction techniques. When attached to cloth these brooches would have looked remarkably similar and only on close inspection would it have been clear that each was unique. Although by reason of the lost-wax casting or hand forging each brooch is unique, the general form of each is highly visually connected to other brooches hinting at their role in advertising connection and similarity. Yet, the differences in each brooch, even when difference was not necessary to form the design, implies a desire to maintain individuality be it indicative of the individual metalworker, or the individual who was adorned with the brooch.

Brooches were favoured for deposition in burials in the Yorkshire Wolds but are otherwise relatively rare in any context further north. In Scotland, before the Late Iron Age, we see continuity of the Bronze Age tradition of dress pins in lieu of, or quite possibly in preference over, brooches (Hunter 2009, 151). These are not the kind of pins which are replicated in brooch form. The same seems also to be true of Ireland (Raftery 1983, 157; Becker 2008). Yet in southern Britain where brooches were more popular, pins are frequently found at the same sites including those that have yielded several brooches such as Cold Kitchen Hill in Wiltshire (Becker 2008; Adams 2013, 234). The presence or absence of brooches then appears to be connected with regional choices, the response of a group or dispersed groups to what the wearing a brooch might or might not mean about their identity.

Brooches are relatively rare finds in graves even in the Middle Iron Age suggesting that either it was not appropriate to bury everyone with a brooch or not everyone had access to a brooch. Mike Parker Pearson has discussed the arguments against equating funerary dress and the contents of graves with simple representations of the dress of the living or the status of the deceased (Parker Pearson 1999, 85). As described above the brooch evidence from burials does not follow a simple pattern: they are not buried with children but may be found with male and female adults of all ages; they occur in simply furnished graves or in more elaborate burials with chariots and other rare and potent items; they may be made from local metals or embellished with exotic materials. Their rarity and materiality suggest these to be objects indicative of status: in this sense status is the ability to obtain rare, finely crafted objects or to have those bestowed upon one. They were expensive items in terms of the resources required to acquire and make the objects and the loss of that item when it was removed from circulation amongst the living. Yet, their varied associations with other indicators of different social position or social role, including gender, age, access to other 'expensive' items and style of burial, means even if we wanted to make the simple equations Parker Pearson argues against, we could not because the evidence just does not fit. For example, although there is a positive association of coral-decorated and ornate bronze brooches with more elaborately furnished graves these are also found in more simple graves and in non-burial contexts (Adams 2013, 157–8, 228–30).

In all likelihood brooches were not objects with a singular role or meaning. The wider patterning visible in the regional and deposition evidence hints at an alternative explanation for the presence or absence of a brooch in a burial and the variable rate at which the quantities of brooches in burials increases over time in different regions highlights changes in the connections drawn between people, their remains and these objects. A brooch as a personal item could reference an individual but its deposition with groups of other brooches or other metalwork could represent that individual's location within a genealogical or social group (e.g. Pryor 2005, 56; Adams 2013, 179–205). As Wells suggests, after Krämer, brooches as fasteners represent 'holding things together' (Wells 2012, 105) the brooch holds either side of the fabric together to keep the individual warm. Although many of the brooches discussed here were not suited to this function, the wearing of a brooch could have made reference to this quality of clasping. This may be further supported by the use of brooches to secure bags containing mirrors as in the Middle Iron Age Wetwang Village chariot burial (Hill 2001), and the Late Iron Age cremation from Chilham Castle, Kent with two brooches possibly clasping the cloth bag and the brooch linked to the handle of the Portesham mirror (Joy 2010, 79–80). Where brooches were deposited *en masse* (as at Grandcourt Farm, Norfolk) they might have had a dual function of representing the individuals who owned the brooches and the group who were being held together by this deposition. However, we should be cautious in applying our own associations of the dual meaning of words to interpret what an Iron Age object signified (Tilley 1989, 185).

Conclusion

The quantity of finds indicates that either very few people owned brooches in the Early and Middle Iron Age or that brooches were carefully kept and rarely discarded. Either way this would indicate that a brooch was a valuable item. They were used by the living and worn by both women and men. These artefacts were important because they were placed where they could be seen on peoples' clothing, on the wrapping of the deceased, or on the wrapping of other items. Clearly we cannot force a single interpretation of the role or relevance of brooches to identity at this time, but we should instead embrace the multiplicity of their differing connections with individuals and with groups. I propose that contra to previous opinion, the rarity of brooches before the Late Iron Age and their relatively ubiquitous nature during it in fact heightens their earlier connection with individuals. Rather than increasing individuality, the frequency of brooches in the Late Iron Age instead standardises people, or places them in particular identity groups. People were already interested in their personal appearance before 150 BC and the change we see in the artefact evidence is less a sign of change in the way people presented themselves and more a change in the way people interacted and connected as a group.

Bibliography

Adams, S. A. (2013) *The First Brooches in Britain: from Manufacture to Deposition in the Early and Middle Iron Age.* Unpublished PhD Thesis, University of Leicester. Available at: http://hdl.handle.net/2381/28593 [accessed March 2016].

Adams, S. (2014) Iron in a time of change: brooch distribution and production in Middle Iron Age Britain. In S. Hornung (ed.) *Produktion, Distribution, Ökonomie. Siedlungs- und Wirtschaftsmuster der Latènezeit. Akten des internationalen Kolloquiums in Otzenhausen 28.-30. Oktober 2011*, 171–87. Bonn, Habelt Verlag.

Adams, S. (2015) Early and Middle Iron Age Bow brooches from Britain. *Later Prehistoric Finds Group Datasheets 1.* Available at: https://sites.google.com/site/laterprehistoricfindsgroup/home/lpfg-datasheets [accessed March 2016].

Adams, S., Booth, A., Haselgrove, C. and Joy, J. (forthcoming) Iron Age brooches, coins and other copper alloy objects from Grandcourt Farm, Middleton, Norfolk. Unpublished report, Archaeological Project Services, Heckington.

Alexander, J. (1973) The study of fibulae (safety pins). In C. Renfrew (ed.) *The Explanation of Culture Change*, 185–94. London, Duckworth.

Allen, L. and Webley, L. (2007) Metalwork. In L. Webley, J. Timby and M. Wilson (2007) *Fairfield Park, Stotfold, Bedfordshire: Later Prehistoric Settlement in the Eastern Chilterns*, 94–6. Bedford, Bedfordshire Archaeological Council (Bedfordshire Archaeology Monograph 7).

Becker, K. (2008) Iron Age ring-headed pins in Ireland, Britain and on the Continent. *Archaeologisches Korrespondenzblatt* 38(4), 513–20.

Bietti Sestieri, A. M. and Macnamara, E. (2007) *Prehistoric Metal Artefacts from Italy (3500-720 BC) in the British Museum.* London, British Museum Press.

Bretz-Mahler, D. (1971) *La Civilisation de La Tène I en Champagne: Le Faciès Marnien.* Paris, Centre National de la Recherche Scientifique.

Brück, J. (2006) Death, exchange and reproduction in the British Bronze Age. *European Journal of Archaeology* 9(1), 73–101.

Brown, F., Howard-Davis, C., Brennand, M., Boyle, A., Evans, T., O'Connor, S., Spence, A., Heawood, R. and Lupton, A., eds. (2007) *The Archaeology of the A1(M) Darrington to Dishforth DBFO Road Scheme*. Lancaster, Oxford Archaeology North (Lancaster Imprints 12).

Champion, S. (1982) Exchange and ranking: the case of coral. In C. Renfrew, C. and S. Shenann (eds.) *Ranking, Resource and Exchange: Aspects of the Archaeology of Early European Society*, 67–72. Cambridge, Cambridge University Press.

Crowfoot, E. (1991) The textiles. In I. M. Stead (ed.) *Iron Age Cemeteries in East Yorkshire: Excavations at Burton Fleming, Rudston, Garton-on-the-Wold and Kirkburn*, 119–25. London, British Museum Press.

Cunliffe, B. and Poole, C. (2000) *The Danebury Environs Programme: The Prehistory of a Wessex Landscape. Volume 2, Part 3: Suddern Farm, Middle Wallop, Hants 1991 and 1996*. Oxford, Institute for Archaeology (Oxford University Committee for Archaeology Monograph 49).

Dent, J. M. (1982) Cemeteries and settlement patterns of the Iron Age on the Yorkshire Wolds. *Proceedings of the Prehistoric Society* 48, 437–57.

Dent, J. (1995) A distinctive form of inlaid brooch from Iron Age Britain. In B. Raftery (ed.) *Sites and Sights of the Iron Age. Essays on Fieldwork and Museum Research presented to Ian Mathieson Stead*, 41–8. Oxford, Oxbow (Oxbow Monograph 56).

Desenne, S., Pommepuy, C. and Demoule, J.-P. (2009) Bucy-le-Long, Aisne. Une nécropole et etudes: une approche de la population, des sépultures et du mobilier. *Revue Archeologique de Picardie*. Numero Spécial 26.

Eckardt, H. (2008) Technologies of the body: Iron Age and Roman grooming and display. In D. Garrow, C. Gosden and J. D. Hill (eds) *Rethinking Celtic Art*, 113–28. Oxford, Oxbow Books.

Evans, T. L. (2004) *Quantitative Identities: A Statistical Summary and Analysis of Iron Age Cemeteries in North-Eastern France 600-130 B.C.* Oxford, Archaeopress (British Archaeological Reports, International Series 1226).

Fitzpatrick, A. P. (1997) *Archaeological Excavations on the Route of the A27 Westhampnett Bypass, West Sussex, 1992. Volume 2: the Cemeteries*. Salisbury, Trust for Wessex Archaeology (Wessex Archaeology Report 12).

Fitzpatrick, A. P. (2007) Dancing with dragons: fantastic animals in the earlier Celtic art of Iron Age Britain. In C. Haselgrove and T. Moore (eds.) *The Later Iron Age in Britain and Beyond*, 341–57. Oxford, Oxbow Books.

Fox, C. (1923) *The Archaeology of the Cambridge Region*. Cambridge, Cambridge University Press.

Fox, C. (1927) A La Tène brooch from Wales: with notes on the typology and distribution of these brooches in Britain. *Archaeologia Cambrensis* 82, 67–112.

Fürst, S. (2010) *Die Südwestdeutschen Korallenfunde der Hallstatt-und Frühlatènezeit im Spiegel Raman-Spektroskopischer Analysen*. Unpublished Masters thesis, Johannes Gutenberg Universität Mainz.

Gell, A. (1998) *Art and Agency: An Anthropological Theory*. Oxford, Clarendon Press.

Giles, M. (2008) Identity, community and the person in later prehistory. In J. Pollard (ed.) *Prehistoric Britain*, 330–50. Oxford, Blackwell.

Giles, M. (2012) *A Forged Glamour. Landscape, Identity and Material Culture in the Iron Age*. Oxford, Windgather Press.

Halkon, P. (2008) *Archaeology and Environment in a Changing East Yorkshire Landscape: the Foulness Valley c. 800 BC to c. AD 400*. Oxford, Archaeopress (British Archaeological Reports, British Series 472).

Hartridge, R. (1978) Excavations at the prehistoric and Romano-British site on Slonk Hill, Shoreham, Sussex. *Sussex Archaeological Collections* 116, 69–141.

Haselgrove, C. (1997) Iron Age brooch deposition and chronology. In A. Gwilt and C. Haselgrove (eds.) *Reconstructing Iron Age Societies. New Approaches to the British Iron Age*, 51–73. Oxford, Oxbow Books (Oxbow Monograph Series 71).

Hattatt, R. (1982) *Ancient and Romano-British Brooches*. Sherborne, Dorset Publishing.

Hattatt, R. (1985) *Iron Age and Roman Brooches*. Oxford, Oxbow Books.

Hattatt, R. (1987) *Brooches of Antiquity. A Third Selection of the Author's Collection*. Oxford, Oxbow Books.

Hattatt, R. (1989) *Ancient Brooches and Other Artefacts. A Fourth Selection of Brooches together with some other Antiquities from the Author's Collection.* Oxford, Oxbow Books.

Herdt, G. (1987) *The Sambia, Ritual and Gender in New Guinea.* New York and London, Holt, Reinhart and Winston.

Hill, J. D. 1995. The Pre-Roman Iron Age in Britain and Ireland (ca. 800 B.C. to A.D. 100). *Journal of World Prehistory* 9(1), 47–98.

Hill, J. D. (2001) Wetwang Village chariot excavation. Unpublished site report, British Museum, BM 2001,0401.19.

Hodson, F. (1964) Cultural groupings within the British pre-Roman Iron Age. *Proceedings of the Prehistoric Society* 30, 99–110.

Hughes, E. G. (1994) An Iron Age barrow burial at Bromfield, Shropshire. *Proceedings of the Prehistoric Society* 60, 395–402.

Hull, M. R. and Hawkes, C. F. C. (1987) *Corpus of Ancient Brooches in Britain: pre-Roman Bow Brooches.* Oxford: British Archaeological Reports (British Archaeological Reports, British Series 168).

Hunter, F. (2009) Miniature masterpieces: unusual Iron Age brooches from Scotland. In G. Cooney, K. Becker, J. Coles, M. Ryan and S. Sievers (eds.) *Relics of Old Decency: Archaeological Studies in Later Prehistory. A Festschrift for Barry Raftery*, 143–55. Dublin, Wordwell.

Joy, J. (2010) *Iron Age Mirrors. A Biographical Approach.* Oxford, Archaeopress (British Archaeological Reports, British Series 518).

Joy, J. (2011) Exploring status and identity in later Iron Age Britain: reinterpreting mirror burials. In L. Armada and T. Moore (eds.) *Western Europe in the First Millennium BC: Crossing the Divide*, 468–87. Oxford, Oxford University Press.

Jundi, S. and Hill, J. D. (1998) Brooches and identities in first century A.D. Britain: more than meets the eye? In C. Forcey, J. G. Hawthorne and R. Witcher (eds.) *TRAC 97. Proceedings of the Seventh Annual Theoretical Roman Archaeology Conference Nottingham 1997*, 125–37. Oxford, Oxbow Books.

Knight, D. (1987) An Early Iron Age hillfort at Castle Yard, Farthingstone, Northamptonshire. *Northamptonshire Archaeologist* 21, 31–40.

Nowakowski, J. A. (1991) Trethellan Farm, Newquay: the excavation of a lowland Bronze Age settlement and Iron Age cemetery. *Cornish Archaeology* 30, 5–242.

Mackreth, D. F. (2011) *Brooches in Late Iron Age and Roman Britain.* Oxford, Oxbow Books.

Marion, S. (2004) *Recherches sur l'âge du Fer en Ile-de-France. Entre Hallstatt final et La Tène finale. Analyse des sites fouillés. Chronologie et société. Volume 1.* Oxford, Archaeopress (British Archaeological Reports, International Series 1231).

Miller, D. (2010) *Stuff.* Cambridge, Polity Press.

Parfitt, K. (1995) *Iron Age Burials from Mill Hill, Deal.* London, British Museum Press.

Parker Pearson, M. (1999) *The Archaeology of Death and Burial.* Stroud, Sutton.

Pryor, F. (2005) *Flag Fen. Life and Death of a Prehistoric Landscape.* Stroud, Tempus.

Raftery, B. (1983) *A Catalogue of Irish Iron Age Antiquities.* Marburg, Veröffentlichung des Vorgeschichtlichen Seminars, Special Volume 1.

Smith, R. (1905) *A Guide to the Antiquities of the Early Iron Age of Central and Western Europe (including the British Late-Keltic Period) in the Department of British and Medieval Antiquities.* London, Trustees of the British Museum.

Smith, R. (1909) Harborough Cave. *Proceedings of the Society of Antiquaries of London (Second Series)* 22, 135–45.

Sofaer Derevenski, J. (2000) Material culture shock: confronting expectations in the material culture of children. In J. Sofaer Derevenski (ed.) *Children and Material Culture*, 3–16. London and New York, Routledge.

Sørensen, M. L. S. (2007) On gender negotiation and its materiality. In S. Hamilton, R. Whitehouse and K. Wright (eds.) *Archaeology and Women: Ancient and Modern Issues*, 41–51. Walnut Creek, Left Coast Press.

Stead, I. M. (1991) *Iron Age Cemeteries in East Yorkshire: Excavations at Burton Fleming, Rudston, Garton-on-the-Wolds and Kirkburn.* London, British Museum Press.

Stead, I. M. and Rigby, V. (1999) *The Morel Collection. Iron Age Antiquities from Champagne in the British Museum.* London, British Museum Press.

Tilley, C. (1989) Interpreting material culture. In I. Hodder (ed.) *The Meanings of Things: Material Culture and Symbolic Expression*, 185–94. London and New York, Routledge.

Wells, P. S. (2008) *Image and Response in Early Europe.* London, Duckworth.

Wells, P. S. (2012) *How Ancient Europeans Saw the World. Vision, Patterns, and the Shaping of the Mind in Prehistoric Times.* Princeton and Oxford, Princeton University Press.

Wheeler, R. E. M. (1943) *Maiden Castle, Dorset.* Oxford, Oxford University Press.

Whitehouse, R. (2007) Gender and archaeology of women: do we need both? In S. Hamilton, R. Whitehouse and K. Wright (eds.) *Archaeology and Women: Ancient and Modern Issues*, 27–40. Walnut Creek, Left Coast Press.

Chapter 4

'Active brooches': theorising brooches of the Roman north-west (first to third centuries AD)

Tatiana Ivleva

Introduction
This chapter provides a survey of the role of brooches as a part of Roman dress by discussing the symbolic nature of these objects of personal adornment. Rather than merely considering brooches as functional dress accessories, this chapter will explore their active role in expressing and creating particular aspects of identity such as ethnicity, gender, status, and age. Brooches worn by all sections of Roman society, including civilian and military individuals, women and men, poor and rich, as well as the rarely discussed demographic of children, will be examined. The focus is on brooches produced and worn in the north-west provinces of the Roman Empire in the period from the first to third centuries AD, with some glances into the earlier and later periods. This will therefore be a broad survey, exploring the plural social role of brooches in the culturally diverse north-west Roman provinces, rather than a fine-grained typological study of the many different brooch types that were available. This chapter also assesses evidence from the Anglophone, German, French and Dutch literature on the subject to provide a broader overview of Roman provincial brooches and why they matter.

Brooches, known in Latin as *fibulae*, were an integral part of clothing in the provincial north-west and occur in their thousands throughout the Empire. Usually made of copper alloy, sometimes of iron and only very occasionally of gold and silver, brooches were produced using various manufacturing techniques, and in a variety of forms, sizes, and decorative styles. In spite of these myriad variables Roman brooches have a number of common features. All brooch types were based on three main forms: bow (brooches arched in profile), plate (flat ones including zoomorphic and skeuomorphic forms), or penannular (open ring-shaped). Similarly, while the sizes of brooches varied, ranging from *c.* 30mm to over 120mm, the majority of brooches on average did not exceed 50–60mm in length or diameter. Manufacturing techniques also differed depending on the material used and the brooch type. Brooches made of iron were wrought, while copper-alloy and sometimes gold and silver ones, were usually cast. Most brooches of the early to mid-first century AD were made from solid metal that had been hammered into shape, compared to brooches of the late first to third centuries AD, which were cast from clay moulds (Bayley and Butcher 2004, 28–9; see also Guillaumet 1984). Brooches that combined wrought and casting techniques and examples made from rolled or folded sheets are also known (Bayley and Butcher 2004, 29; Mackreth 2011, 4). The casting technique allowed brooches to be manufactured quickly and provided the ability to reproduce the same types of brooches on a mass scale. Variety also existed in ways that their surfaces were decorated. To add colour to the yellowish surface of copper-alloy brooches, enamel (powdered glass) was fused to the metal. For brooches to appear silvery, tinning could be applied (Mackreth 2011, 5). The majority of bow and plate brooches dating to the late first to second centuries AD were decorated in these ways, though the types produced and worn in the mid- to late third century were more often gilded and had glass or stone settings. Regardless of the chronological period, other decorative features such as application of dots, triangles, and silver wires are known, and even figures of animals that were fitted into a slot on the brooch head.

The first and foremost function for any brooch was to hold two pieces of a person's clothing together: usually outer garments like cloaks were pinned to tunics. There is sufficient pictorial evidence of people wearing brooches, particularly representations on tombstones, to indicate that brooches were positioned on the upper part of the costume that covered the torso/chest area. Because they functioned as clothes-fasteners, men and women alike wore brooches in nearly every province of the north-west Roman Empire, though differences in custom may have existed according to gender (for discussion see below). Their primary function, which was to fasten clothes, was linked to a secondary function: decoration (Allason-Jones 2005, 121). The brooch's position at shoulder and chest levels, a highly visible place, and various decorative techniques, suggest that brooches were worn to be seen. Moreover, although only one and sometimes two brooches were actually needed to connect two pieces of clothing together, a third and even a fourth brooch were sometimes added for purely non-functional purposes. Some brooch types were only used for decoration, as is suggested by the small length of the pin and/or the small gap between the pin and catch plate on some examples, which would not accommodate a sufficient amount of fabric to fasten a thick woollen cloaks effectively (Allason-Jones 2013, 27–8; Fillery-Travis 2012, 135). The ornamental potential of a brooch was therefore 'fully appreciated and exploited' by the population, making them more than 'purely utilitarian object[s]' (Johns 1996, 147).

The archaeological record shows that brooches occur in a variety of contexts, turning up in settlements, cemeteries, sanctuaries, hoards and other ritual deposits. The significance of these contexts is discussed in the following section of this chapter, but here it is important to note that as integral parts of Roman dress, brooches were used in various ways, and were not only worn on a daily basis. The choice of type, style and/or form would have varied depending on the circumstances in which these objects were used. This choice indicates that people sought to communicate particular messages about their positions, affinities, and preferences through wearing, depicting, and depositing brooches. This indicates the existence of a third function of brooches as signifiers of identity. The recognition that 'brooches are more than meets the eye' in the Late Iron Age and in Roman Europe was promoted by Jundi and Hill (1998) in their article of the same title. They stated that a brooch can no longer be used as 'just another archaeological artefact' but should be seen as 'a communicative tool allowing different types of identities to be expressed or created' (Jundi and Hill 1998, 136). Brooches are therefore now regarded not only as functional tools used to secure clothing or as decorative tools to adorn dress, but also as active participants in constructing, manipulating or renegotiating the identities of their wearers, owners, and makers.

Brooches and identities: to pin or not to pin?

Compared with other objects of personal adornment, brooches have always stood out in their popularity among archaeologists. They are frequently and quickly identifiable during excavation or field walking due to their recognisable shape. Their popularity and abundance has led to brooches becoming the subject of numerous detailed studies compared to other artefacts of personal adornment. The number of works published on Roman brooches in any modern language is hard to count, though a few major studies, that have become standard reference works, deserve a special mention. For British evidence these are the volumes by Bayley and Butcher (2004), Mackreth (2011), Snape (1993) and Swift (2000) on the fourth-century crossbow brooches; in German see *Fibel und Fibeltracht* (2011), Heynowski (2012) and Völling (1994); and in French see Dollfus (1973), Feugère (1985) and Philippe (1999). In spite of well over half a century of scholarly research into brooch typology, style, design, distribution and dating, only relatively recently have brooches begun to be studied with more sophisticated theoretical approaches in mind. After Jundi and Hill's (1998) seminal article the concept of identity has become attached to all aspects of brooch use. The focus has therefore shifted from the typological development of different brooch types and their distribution, to the social significance of brooches as identity markers (*cf.* the meeting and proceeding of '*Fibulae* in the Roman Empire' (FIRE) group, Grabherr, Kainrath and Schierl 2013, also works of Booth 2015; Callewaert 2012; Collins 2010; Curta 2005; Eckardt 2005; Edgar 2012; Fillery-Travis 2012; Harrison 1999; Heeren 2014; Hunter 2008; 2010; Ivleva 2011; McIntosh 2010 and 2011; Pudney 2011).

The prominence of identity as a theme can be connected with the growing number of studies with a focus on this subject (Pitts 2007, 693). In the course of Roman provincial studies, often fuelled by discussion surrounding the redefinition or abandonment of the term 'Romanisation' (on the debate see Hingley 2005; Schörner

2005; Mattingly 2004; 2011; Gardner 2013), a theoretical and conceptual vacuum was created as identity started to be regarded as a substitute and synonym for the 'R-word' (on the critique of the identity paradigm see Brubaker and Cooper 2000; Gardner 2013; Pitts 2007; Revell 2009; Rothe 2012a; Versluys 2014). The popularity of identity had led to its being studied for its own sake (Insoll 2007, 4; Pitts 2007, 693) with research mainly dealing with cataloguing various types of identities and the ways they can be determined in the archaeological record. Shortcomings also lie in terminology: modern theoretical applications pollute our understanding of past identities (Insoll 2007, 4; Meskell 2007, 32; Pitts 2007, 699–700). What is understood by, for instance, age identity might not have been of any importance to people in the past, and instead it may have been understood as an expression of what is known today as gender identity (Hodos 2010, 18; Pitts 2007, 700). In studies discussing brooches, identity has come to be seen as a tool to analyse many facets of the plural functions of brooches. Most would now say that brooches are indicative of a number of identities, such as gender, status, age, social status, and ethnicity.

Therefore, the term identity has been somewhat overused in Roman provincial studies, and some researchers have voiced their concerns that we need to move beyond it (Casella and Fowler 2005; Pitts 2007). A more flexible model that has come forward recently is to analyse the experiences of agents and their actions through social practices, therefore shifting the focus from identification to experience (Meskell 2007, 30; Pitts 2007, 701). Here, identity is seen as being created through the social interactions of an individual person (self) with their surroundings (the other), and that these social interactions produce norms and rules for that individual to follow or reject (Eckardt 2014, 4; Rowlands 2007, 68; *cf.* also Brather 2009; Diaz-Andreu and Lucy 2005; Jones 1997; Rowlands 2007; Versluys forthcoming). In other words, the inner self is influenced by outside interventions and confrontations with 'the other', a struggle through which identity is born. This model does not diminish the importance of identity, since identity becomes a medium where 'self' and 'other' interrelate (Gardner 2007, 18). Rather it provides a new dimension to our understanding of how an individual person attends to and experiences the world through material objects by moving the point of study to the level of an individual, or his or her inner self (Eckardt 2014, 4).

Regarding brooches, following Pitts' (2007) argument that the patterns of use and contexts reflect the social and cultural changes in any given society, attention should be devoted to exploring the multifaceted brooches and their multiple uses in a variety of social and cultural contexts rather than pinning down what kind of identities these objects project, construct, negotiate or negate. The discussion should therefore start with acknowledging the motivations that guided individuals to choose a particular brooch and their strategies to involve that brooch in the processes of self-expression, including the construction or negotiation of identities that were by-products of these actions (paraphrasing Fowler 2004, 4 on the importance of studies of selfhood).

The discovery of Roman brooches in a variety of archaeological contexts reveals that their purposes were not limited to being dress accessories, to fastening garments or being identity markers. Considering the multivocal nature of material culture (Derks 2009, 241), individuals experienced brooches in various ways and responded to that by giving brooches particular values. Brooches fulfilled the role of objects of desire, commodities for exchange and gift giving, items of fashion, holders of memory, and suitable accompaniments of the dead as I have argued elsewhere and as will be briefly discussed below (Ivleva 2012; 2016). They facilitated various mind-sets such as hope and familiarity, joy and mourning, comfort and discomfort (Turkle 2007). The pluralism of types, manufacturing methods and decorative techniques indicate that brooches can be seen as containers of creativity and visionary art. Thus, brooches may have been engaged in the process of negotiating a variety of selfhoods, world experiences, identity expressions, and cultural and artistic encounters.

Brooches have been recovered from hoards and sacred sites throughout the Roman north-west (van Impe and Creemers 2002, 47; Johns 2002, 74–5; Pulles and Roymans 1994; Pudney 2011, 123–6). In Roman Gaul and Britain brooches appear to have been particularly popular votive objects, and are found on many sites associated with ritual activity (for the French evidence see among others Canny and Dilly 1997; Devillers 2000; Fauduet and Pommeret 1985; Vodoz 1983; for the British evidence see Butcher 1977 and 1986, 319, note 80; Simpson and Blance 1998). This treatment of objects primarily used as accessories and decorations implies changes in the value and meaning of brooches, from secular to sacred, or from active to non-active. By way of contrast, the occurrence of brooches in rubbish pits indicates their non-value, i.e., after fulfilling the purpose of decoration and pinning garments together they were no longer needed and were thrown away. However, what some may see as rubbish thrown away during the abandonment of a site, others may re-evaluate: brooches and other objects of domestic use may have been deliberately abandoned and ritually deposited (Jundi and Hill 1998, 128–9; Pudney 2011, 121–2). All three contexts (votive, hoard and rubbish) imply the death of active usage, whereby brooches were taken out of circulation and were intentionally refused their primary functional purpose. In each case, the symbolism of 'killing' the object plays on different levels; high symbolic meaning may have been at stake for brooches given away as votive offerings, and low or no meaning might have been attached to brooches thrown away in rubbish pits. For brooches that occurred in hoards the value may have depended on the nature of the deposit. In votive hoards, purposefully deposited without any intention of a later recovery, brooches may have high emblematic value. This is demonstrated by two elaborately designed silver-gilt brooches of a type known as trumpet brooches found as part of the votive hoard near modern village of Backworth in England, apparently buried as gifts to the mother goddesses (Johns 1996, 211–13). In cases when brooches were deliberately buried in the ground with the intention to retrieve them later, high (economic) value may have been associated with them; this is especially valid for brooches made of precious metals such as silver and gold, richly decorated with incised patterns or silver wires and inlays. An example comes from a Roman coin hoard found in Knustford area of Cheshire in England containing amongst other things three cast silver-gilt brooches of the trumpet style decorated with elaborate incised patterns (Knustford area hoard, see Portable Antiquities Scheme Nos. LVPL-180D95, LVPL-9BCE31, LVPL-B9E875; on another hoard with brooches found nearby see Abdy et al. 2004). Brooches appearing in hoards may have been used to fasten wrappings containing precious objects, in such cases, the brooch's primary purpose was revived.

Another way brooches enter the archaeological record is through casual loss. In many cases, brooches seem to appear in the context of roadsides or fields, places without a site or any site nearby, or beneath the floor of a building, where no other objects were found. They also appear on Roman battlefields, where they may have been lost during battle or after at a time of looting (Ball 2014, 97). Brooches could be lost without the owner noticing. Some pin mechanisms, in particular hinged ones, are less secure meaning they tend to fail more often causing the brooch to fall into a difficult to reach place (see Adams this volume).

Brooches were also frequently deposited in cremation burials across the Roman north-west (Philpott 1991; 1993 and Pollock 2006 for British evidence; Heeren 2014 for Dutch evidence; Faider-Feytmans 1965 for French evidence; Laet et al. 1972 for Belgic evidence). Although some brooches were included as grave goods or were used to pin together wrappings containing the cremated bone, others were placed in ditches outside the grave, perhaps after the burial had taken place or during the funeral feast (Heeren 2014, 444–5, 447). A significant number of brooches would have entered the cremation assemblage as part of the clothing worn by the deceased when they were placed on the funeral pyre. It has been determined through various experiments that copper-alloy brooches can only be partially damaged in funeral pyres rather than completely burned, since the melting point of copper alloy is over 1000°C and open-air cremation fires burn at a much lower heat (Edgar 2012, 108 with further literature). Yet, only rarely in archaeological reports is fire damage to a brooch recorded (Edgar 2012, 157), so it is difficult to determine in each particular case the way in which a brooch ended up in a cremation burial. Nevertheless, it shows that relatives of the deceased had various choices in how to include brooches and each act could have had a special significance, through which various forms of communally constructed, perceived or idealised identities could have been projected and communicated (Heeren 2014, 454–5; Parker Pearson 1999).

The aspects of pinning, decorating and symbolising suggest a passive role for brooches: individuals choose from this repertoire an action that suits their purposes. Indeed brooches have the capacity to act in a way that agents choose for them, but they are also active participants in shaping agents, their selfhood and their identities that are constructed through social interactions. One speaks of a mutual dependence in human-object relationships, where artefacts define humans and humans define artefacts (Hodder 2012, especially 27–39 and 64–87). In this approach to material culture it is acknowledged that humans create brooches and choose actions for them (passive role), but that brooches also create humans (active role). The active role of brooches is reflected in their everyday role in constructing the social realities of agents. Following the idea of object agency (Gell 1998; Hodder 2011 and 2012), brooches are regarded here not as representational objects, but as having a form of agency: through the particular effects they have on those who create and use them, brooches may influence humans to act in particular ways. It should be taken into account that a brooch's agency moves beyond an animist approach in seeing artefacts as having a soul or being alive, or having an actant identity (Ingold 2007; Latour 2005). Agency here is simply a by-product of a brooch's physicality. This approach allows us to move away from the question of what brooches mean or symbolise to asking what brooches do. It creates a new avenue for exploring how brooches provided a repertoire of actions for individuals to articulate their everyday realities, and create their selfhood and socially influenced identities. What these actions are will be explored in the next section.

What brooches do and how they do it

The aim of this section is to address what brooches do (Fig. 4.1) and outline the repertoire of actions that entangle humans with brooches. The actions of pinning and decorating have been already briefly discussed in the introduction, and therefore will not again be defined in this section.

Artefacts are like chameleons, which, while staying within the same body, adapt their skin colour and pattern accordingly to variable conditions and situations (Tilley 2004). The shape, colour, and size of a brooch is variable in relation to light or shade, and the position, posture, or movement of the observer and owner (after Ingold 2007, 14 on the changing nature of the surface of a stone in various conditions). These material qualities that are changeable according to context may awaken and stimulate various sensory, sensual and emotional responses in the wearers and viewers. Objects as extensions of human ideas and actions are intertwined with human cognition but also contest and accelerate affective responses (Malafouris and Renfew 2010, 8; also Turkle 2007). Thus, the brooch's visual, colourful, and decorative qualities may have guided human actions towards particular responses such as evocation, provocation, adoration, and so on. These qualities may have also been enhanced by being worn alongside other highly symbolic and semantic canvases such as the dress itself (Harlow 2012). Brooches might therefore be regarded as triggers of various responses.

Brooches also acted as tokens of non-verbal communication. A brooch's visual dominance may have allowed them to act like a badge, signalling affiliations and preferences in the individual's status, profession, religion, politics, ethnicity, and gender (Jundi and Hill 1998, 131). The choice of a particular type of brooch can be regarded as an act of self-expression and a negotiation of socially constructed identities. However, it should be taken into account that brooches acting as badges may be forced onto the individual to wear rather than being a deliberate choice in which a person's preferences were projected (Flowers 2011, 28).

Most brooches may have had a number of owners in their lives, and they may also have travelled as personal accessories of their owners to the edges of the Roman

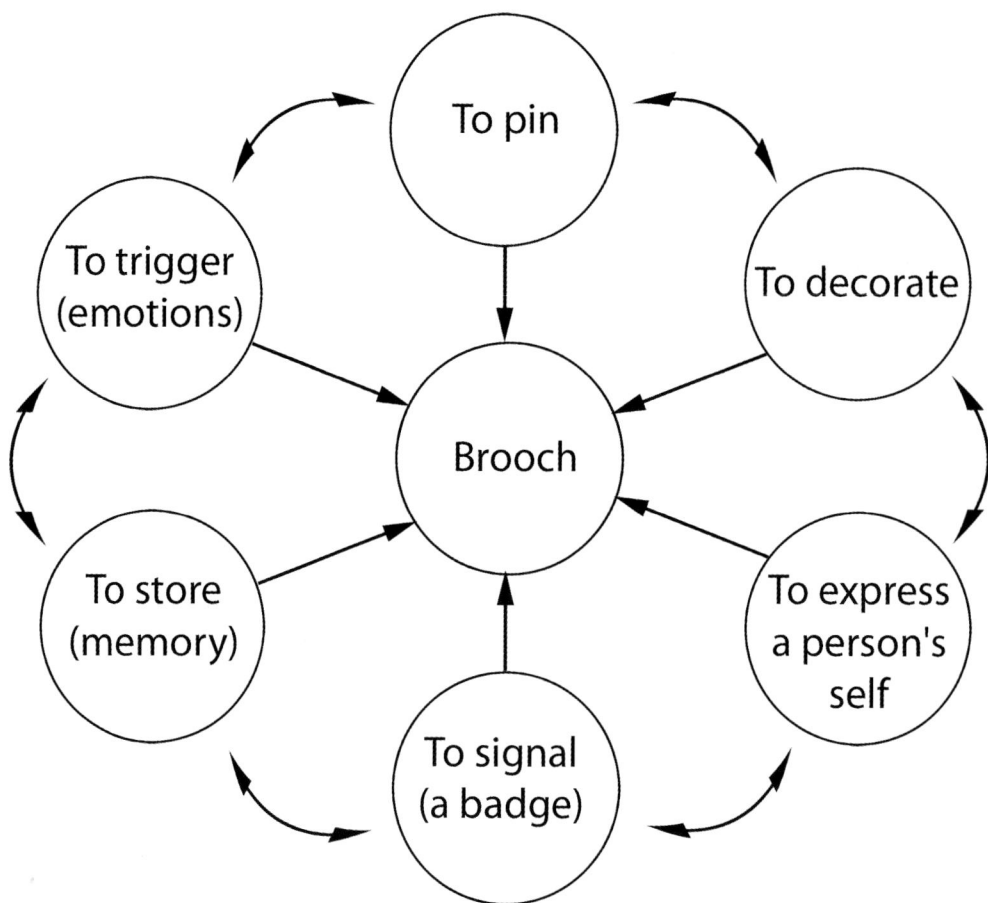

Fig. 4.1: *What brooches do in the Roman north-west (inspired by Brather 2009, 5, fig. 3: Functions of clothes in the Early Modern period; ©Joep van Rijn).*

world. Some also had long histories, which can be partially determined by signs of wear and repair (von Richthofen 1998). This travelling through space and time is akin to the idea of 'object biography' introduced by Kopytoff (1986). Artefacts go through various stages of interpretation, assessment and usage, emerging in different social and cultural spheres. At each stage, they are supplemented or imbued with a new narrative, acquiring new biographies and associations (Hahn and Weiss 2013). Brooches as repositories of past histories and associations, and at the same time acting as bearers of memory, can be exemplified by examples used as heirlooms, cherished and valued for their ancestral associations and connections with the past (Gilchrist 2013, 237–41). Brooches can therefore act as a metaphorical storage of memory, associations, feelings and past activities. This point can be exemplified by finds of brooches in children's graves, which will be discussed below.

All these actions of pinning, storing, decorating, expressing, signalling and triggering do not happen in isolation but occur simultaneously. Brooches that were valued by their owners for their decorative qualities or physical superiority (e.g. a spring or pin that never breaks) may have held particular evocative associations as well as signalled a position within the social reality (*cf.* Gilchrist 2013, 378 on heirlooms). Gender, ethnic or status associations may have worked together with the brooch's physicality to produce a multidimensional representation of an owner's personhood, who, by wearing a consciously chosen brooch, may have triggered particular emotions in the viewers (e.g. 'the others'), therefore contributing to the construction of the social person and identities (as in Fowler 2004, 4).

This interconnectedness between the different active roles of brooches is linked fundamentally to their multiple functions, signifying the pluralistic '*Funktionswandel*' of these objects. The *Funktionswandel* concept can be understood in terms of the conceptualised and contextualised mobility of functions and meanings (Hofmann and Schreiber 2011, 170). People used brooches as a medium for the expression of personhood and the construction of self- and body-awareness in myriad ways and in a variety of social and cultural contexts by constantly changing and adapting brooch uses and meanings according to context and personal wishes. *Funktionswandel* is embedded in the pragmatic and selective nature of humans, who may use, for instance, chopsticks to eat but also as hairpins. For brooches this conceptualised and contextualised mobility can be seen in the following example of drifting associations. As is evident from various studies that will be discussed in detail below, while some brooches were worn exclusively by women to underline and enhance feminine associations, in another community the very same brooches would be undone from their feminine aspects and intentionally ritualised and embedded with sacred meaning (Böhme-Schönberger 2008; Grane 2013; Hunter 2013a; Swift 2003).

What follows now are some preliminary ideas and observations related to brooch use and *Funktionswandel* in various media and contexts in the Roman north-west. I hope also to demonstrate through the concept of *Funktionswandel* how correlating brooches with particular type of identity can be misleading, as the same brooch types appeared to be associated with multiple identities that varied across the space and time in the Roman North-west. The concept of brooches as active agents and *Funktionswandel* provide the necessary tools to understand and outline the workings of the multivocal nature of material culture. Therefore, while the two concepts are the focus of this contribution, they are used more as an illustration of the plurality of functions, and the conceptualised and contextualised mobility of any personal accessories, jewellery items and other artefacts.

'Sexless' brooches, or do brooches have a gender?

Both gender and sex are constructed categories. Diaz-Andreu (2005) and Meskell (2007) see gender as a category built upon culturally perceived sexual differences, which are primarily based on the physical and genetic elements of the body. However, since the writings of Butler (1993), who questioned the pre-determined gendered nature of sex, both gender and sex are also seen as a performance and not limited to static divisions between males and females. Thus, humans may hold a number of possible genders (Diaz-Andreu 2005, 15), as well as qualify their bodily performances in many possible ways within cultural norms (Butler 1993, 2–3). Gender is governed by the socially imposed artificial categories and expectations of the society that defines it, whilst sex is the expression of the inner 'un-subjected' personhood (Butler 1993, 3 calls it 'abject beings'). This flexibility of gender and sex adds further complexities to understanding the 'genderless' and 'sexless' nature of the brooches.

Allason-Jones (1995) discusses the 'sexless' nature of brooches. Taking physicality into account, brooches themselves are indeed 'sexless', unless one considers them as agents with their own inner self (Olsen 2010). At the moment of their creation, brooches do not have any gender associations but are rather given such connotations by human agents. The issue here is that this imposed gender is rather obscure for archaeologists to determine. Pearce (2011, 237–8, 241) in his analysis of funerary rituals in Roman Britain notes that while some remains of the deceased in burials offered a chance to be sexed osteologically, no or low difference in gender associations for artefacts such as brooches was detected. Gender can also be interlinked with other identities. What can be regarded by contemporary researchers as an indicator of gender may equally have constructed other identities such as age or status. An example of this comes from another chronological period and geographical area, namely seventh-century Greece, which is worth noting to show that the *Funktionswandel* of brooches is not confined to the Roman north-west. 'Slavic' bow brooches, exclusively worn by women in Greece, were assumed to express feminine identity, but research by Curta (2005) has shown that that these brooches had little to do with expressions of womanhood, but were rather status-specific and associated with power these women held in society (*cf.* also Pohl 1998).

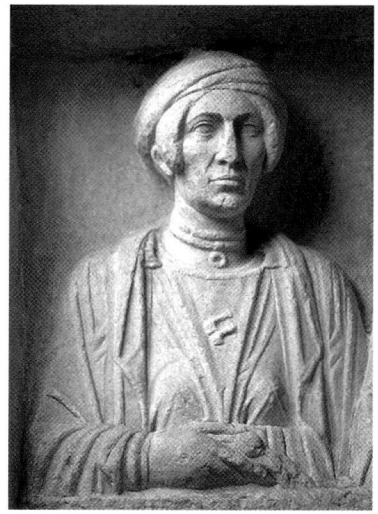

Fig. 4.2: A depiction of a woman wearing four brooches: two Doppelknopffibeln pinning the dress at the shoulders and two knee brooches worn at the centre of the dress. Found in Neumarkt im Tauchental, Austria (Lupa 448-B3; © Ortolf Harl 1998).

For the Roman north-west, the general assumption is that the male style was to wear one brooch, which fastened the cloak on the right shoulder, while the female custom was to wear two or more brooches, where two fastened the dress at both shoulders, and others, usually positioned in the centre of a dress, were used to pin the undertunic to the overtunic (Croom 2002). This is evident from depictions on funerary monuments (Fig. 4.2).

Wearing brooches in pairs seems to have been a female custom, since no tombstone from the Roman Empire depicts men wearing them in this fashion (Allason-Jones 1995, 24; Rothe 2012b, 236). The pictorial evidence is supported in some regions by the archaeological evidence. For instance, early Roman depictions of women on funerary monuments from the lands inhabited by the tribe of the *Treveri* (contemporary Rhine-Moselle region, Germany) corresponds to brooch finds in burials (Rothe 2012b, 236). Women depicted wearing outer tunics with their fabric held by matching pairs of brooches and grave finds from the region support this image (Rothe 2012b, 236; *cf.* also Leifeld 2007). However, the wearing of brooches in pairs did not necessarily only indicate gender or womanhood (Allason-Jones 1995, 24; 2005, 121; Johns 1996, 149). As exemplified by Curta above, other identities may have been projected alongside this, status being one of them.

Particular brooch types have long been associated with the male gender. *Drahtfibel* (with wire bows), knee, penannular and P-shaped brooches have all been linked to the Roman military (Fig. 4.3; McIntosh 2011, 159, after Bayley and Butcher 2004, 179, and Snape 1993, 20; Heynowski 2012, 72: '*Soldatenfibel*'). Knee brooches are especially often referred to as soldier's brooches: they are predominantly found on Roman military forts of the second century in north-west Europe, and their distribution follows the line of the north-west Roman frontier (Allason-Jones 2013, 27 after Cool 1983 and

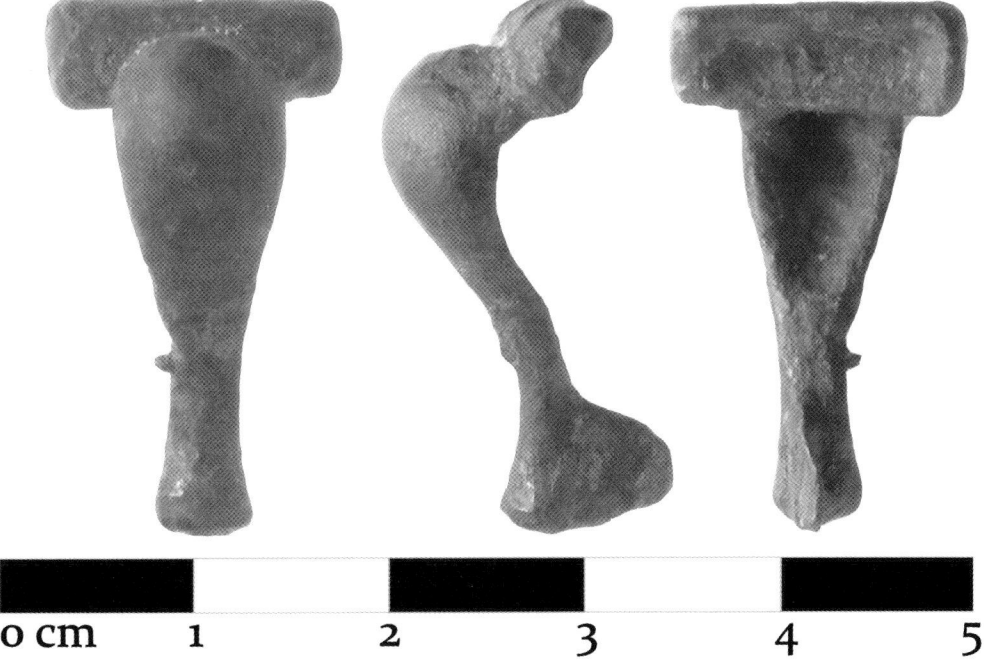

Fig. 4.3: Knee brooch, found in Leeds. PAS Nr. SWYOR-AFCBB2 (PAS finds reproduced under Creative Commons Share-Alike Agreement).

Eckardt 2005). Envisioning this type as a typically male artefact does not, however, work for the whole of the Roman world, as one particular image of a woman shows us (Fig. 4.2). She is depicted wearing what looks like two knee brooches positioned at the centre of her dress (*cf.* also Lupa Nr. 1487 and Nr. 1719. Allason-Jones 2013, 27). Can it mean that women wearing a pair of soldier's brooches were soldier's wives, therefore associating knee brooches with a particular social position within society? This is difficult to answer since the inscription, plausibly identified to accompany the image, tells us that the woman was the wife of a (wealthy) citizen rather than of a serviceman in the Roman army (CIL III 5056 and CIL III 10937).

Such images provoke another question, which is whether in different Roman provinces the same brooch types were purchased by individuals according to personal taste, and if there was little to stop anyone from acquiring brooches from other territories (Allason-Jones 1995, 24). It seems to be the case that the objects' mobility (with owners, traders or as souvenir trinkets) influenced the appropriation of new gendered constructions or the un-doing of existing gender associations once they were taken out of their indigenous milieu (Allison 2013, 75–6). The research of Böhme-Schönberger (1994; 2002; 2008) into the distribution of *Kragen-* and *Distelfibeln* (collared and thistle-shaped brooches) shows that thistle-shaped brooches, for example, were originally worn predominantly by 'Gallic' women on over-garments, but were adopted by 'Germanic' men to become purely male accessories. Collared brooch types in the first phase of their existence in the late La Tène (first century BC) and the pre-Roman period were worn by both men and women but became a popular dress accessory for women in the Augustan period (late first century BC to early first century AD). This shows how brooches can easily be imbued with a gender narrative, moving from genderless associations to objects connected with female or male constructions.

The shape of brooches does not give us a clue as to whether they were predominantly female or male artefacts. Allison (2013, 74) justifiably argues that brooches with bowed or raised profiles used to fasten bulky woollen outer garments were worn by both men and women to fasten their cloaks and tunics. However, the depiction of brooches on tombstones and other sculptural reliefs of the first to third centuries in the Roman north-west shows us that it was predominantly men who wore brooches depicted as round or oval discs with a raised central rosette or a central stone, glass or cameo setting (Fig. 4.4; Croom 2002, 73; *cf.* Lupa Nr. 2978, 10796, 13284, 17644 among many others; *cf.* Allason-Jones 2013, 25 'It is only the image of the emperors that show brooches [in the form of] a disc holding [a] cloak'). In the fourth century, images of brooches change and largely feature the so-called crossbow brooches of the Late Antique period. Crossbow brooches became synonymous with membership of the Roman army or administration, being worn exclusively by high-status, male military and civilian officials (Collins 2010, Swift 2000, 230–1).

It has been generally assumed that the P-shaped type was the predecessor of the crossbow brooch, used and worn predominantly by men associated with the Roman army or in other positions of authority. Yet, considering what has been said about disc brooches above, one may suggest that the crossbow brooch as a status symbol had as its predecessor the *depiction* of the sharply gendered disc brooch on the High Roman Empire sculptural reliefs. In other words, masculinity, wealth, status and power may have been associated with such conventional images of disc brooches, which were considered to be an appropriate emblem for a power representation, while in everyday reality, it did not strictly matter who would wear disc brooches, or when they might.

All this clearly shows the problems of assuming a correlation between a particular individual and a gender, and suggests that brooches might be unhelpful when it comes to identifying the constructed gender of an individual. The brooch's 'conceptualised and contextualised mobility' prevent us from pinpointing feminine or masculine associations, albeit that one should not forget about the strongly gendered crossbow brooch, which was indeed used only by high status men. Our challenge is identifying when particular brooch types, forms, designs or customs of wear were imbued with new gender narratives or became removed from such associations in particular communities, while at the same time being aware of the fact that constructed genders and sexes were in constant flux.

Ethnic connotations

Some brooch types are assumed to have been indicators of ethnicity: restricted to a certain areas and possibly produced and worn almost exclusively by members of particular tribal entities (on the *Flügelfibel* as a Pannonian type, see Láng 1919; on the *Doppelknopf-* and *Flügelfibel* as a Norico-Pannonian type, see Garbsch 1965; on the *Kragenfibel* as a Treveran type, see Böhme-Schönberger 1994). Yet, brooches in their materiality are non-ethnic. Rather, they are products of craftspeople, working with imagery, forms and designs accepted in their social surroundings. The research of Frances McIntosh into the development and distribution of the Romano-British Wirral brooch shows that this type was part of a disposable local consumer culture rather than a deliberate sign of ethnic affiliation (McIntosh 2010; 2013). To this end, such categories as Norico-Pannonian brooches, or specifically Celtic style dragonesque brooches become extremely slippery notions (for the deconstruction of these ideas see Rothe 2013 and Hunter 2010, consequently). Hunter (2013b, 271) notes that what we describe as a Celtic style of a dragonesque brooch may have been seen as a frontier style in the Roman period and perceived as a badge of someone living in the proximity of the military zone rather than a deliberate evocation of indigenous identity.

The notion of a Romano-British brooch should be seen in a similar way. While it can be understood as a pure hybrid of Roman and British art traditions and forms, one must take into account that these brooches were actually a result of cultural mixtures, a combination of Roman, Continental, British and local-British craftsmanship, which were produced within mixed cultural conditions. In this sense, these Romano-British brooches were therefore hybrids of hybrids from their very inception. The problem here is that one cannot perceive 'Roman' or 'British' as fixed taxonomic entities

(Brather 2009; Revell 2009). They were were fragmented and complex notions imbued with multileveled meanings, where being Roman (or British) was always different (Revell 2009; Ivleva 2012). By understanding them more as artefacts made in Britain (i.e. as products of the province of Roman Britain, which was a part of the 'globalised' Roman Empire 'koine'), one can avoid the problems associated with connecting particular artefacts with invented cultural categories (see Hofmann and Schreiber 2011, 171, notes 9 and 10 for further discussion).

Wearing a brooch produced in a particular regional or 'ethnic' style does not necessarily make its owner or wearer a member of this particular ethnic or regional entity. We must take into account that sometimes choices were limited to what was available for purchase from the itinerant craftspeople. For example, in Roman Britain the evidence for the existence of actual workshops which produced brooches of the same type *en masse* is rather small, which suggests brooch manufacture was carried out by either travelling artisans or individual craftspeople working for a small market (Bayley and Butcher 2004, 35–40; Butcher 1977, 42; Mackreth 2011, 242). Therefore, if someone was passing through a particular territory when his or her brooch's pin broke, and there was no possibility to repair it, the wearer may have decided to buy a brooch, manufactured by such a craftsperson. Moreover, if one was living on a site for a longer period of time (for instance, the wives of Roman auxiliary soldiers or traders with branches in different territories), one may have grown accustomed to wearing local dress accessories, although by simply wearing them, he or she might never have become ethnically associated with the community producing them. Another issue here is the nature of ethnicity itself, which constantly shifts, and can be constructed, manipulated or/and multi-layered (Brather 2004; Jones 1997; Lucy 2005). A person may have multi-layered ethnic identities, with each layer being expressed at a particular time through a particular medium in a particular set of circumstances, allowing the various ethnic affiliations to be switched on or off (Wallace-Hadrill 2007, 356–7).

The assumption that brooches in general were used as symbols to deliberately emphasise ethnic origin can be contested. Yet, as shown above, the mobility of objects through time and space allows for them to become imbued with a variety of narratives. My own research on the distribution of British-made brooches in continental Europe suggested that, since they were British products, brooches were symbols associated with a British past (Ivleva 2011; 2012). While in their materiality brooches did not themselves have any British connotations, it is through their encounter with agents that they were given such British narratives. Through wearing a brooch, different messages could have been sent by the owner, including the imposed British narrative that resonated together with all their other meanings and narratives. The brooch's visual appeal may have prompted some people to ask questions regarding where the owner had purchased such an object. The owner, therefore, could have replied that 'he served as a soldier in Britain' or '(s)he travelled to Britain and returned safely' or '(s)he was born in Britain'. Different meanings are emphasised in each case, but a connection with Britain is present in all of them. This 'British-ness' does not necessarily imply ethnic associations; rather, different British pasts as a soldier, a trader or a traveller are emphasised. This suggestion is based on the 'material resonance' theory of Antonaccio, where objects 'do not always retain their original meaning when recontextualised'. However, some of them 'may still retain particular resonance for their users' (Antonaccio 2009, 35). To this end, British-made brooches on the Continent were the sums of material resonances that were doing and undoing their owners' ethnic and past narratives.

Questions left unanswered

Brooches 'made to order'

An issue that has not received much attention from scholars is the extent to which first- to third-century brooches were status- and wealth-related objects. This is of course invalid for the crossbow brooches of the late third to fourth centuries, since they have always been seen in this way. Only recently has Allason-Jones (2013, 28) put forward the question as to whether it is possible to identify brooch types specifically made for the not-so-wealthy members of the Roman provincial society. Brooches produced in gold and silver with a high level of technical expertise may have belonged to rich owners, although Allason-Jones warns that 'wealthy' does not necessarily stand for high status. Wealthy slaves and freedmen are such examples (Allason-Jones 2013, 28).

Hunter (2013b, 273) has shown that inhabitants of military and urban sites in Roman Britain had a particular taste for enamelled brooches, whilst in rural areas relief-decorated brooches were in fashion. While Hunter (2013b, 273) sees this as differences in the visual world of urban versus rural dwellers, it may have also been dependent on the financial possibility to acquire enamelled brooches or access to technology. Enamelling is complex and a substantial amount of time and skill is required to form the cells, fill them with coloured glass or powdered glassy substance, and finally to fire them and fuse the glass to the bronze (Bayley and Butcher 2004, 46–50; Butcher 1977, 41; Fillery-Travis 2012, 154; *cf.* also Bateson and Hedges 1975). This production technique may have been costly and time consuming, resulting in higher prices for enamelled brooches, especially the ones with juxtaposed blocks of enamel of more than two alternating colours (Fig. 4.4; on the amount of working hours required to produce some types see von Richthofen 1998, 244 with further literature).

It is possible that some brooches were actually made to order, where the customers had more influence on the final appearance of a brooch to make it more appropriate for their social position. That local demand played a significant role in brooch supply is exemplified by the persistence of particular brooch types with specific designs from Roman-period sites in Scotland. Consumers preferred objects that fitted their taste, although this has nothing to do with their position in a community but rather with overall communal preferences (Hunter 2013b, 275–6). Some brooches do appear to be customised and specifically adapted to appear more luxurious (*cf.* an Alcester type

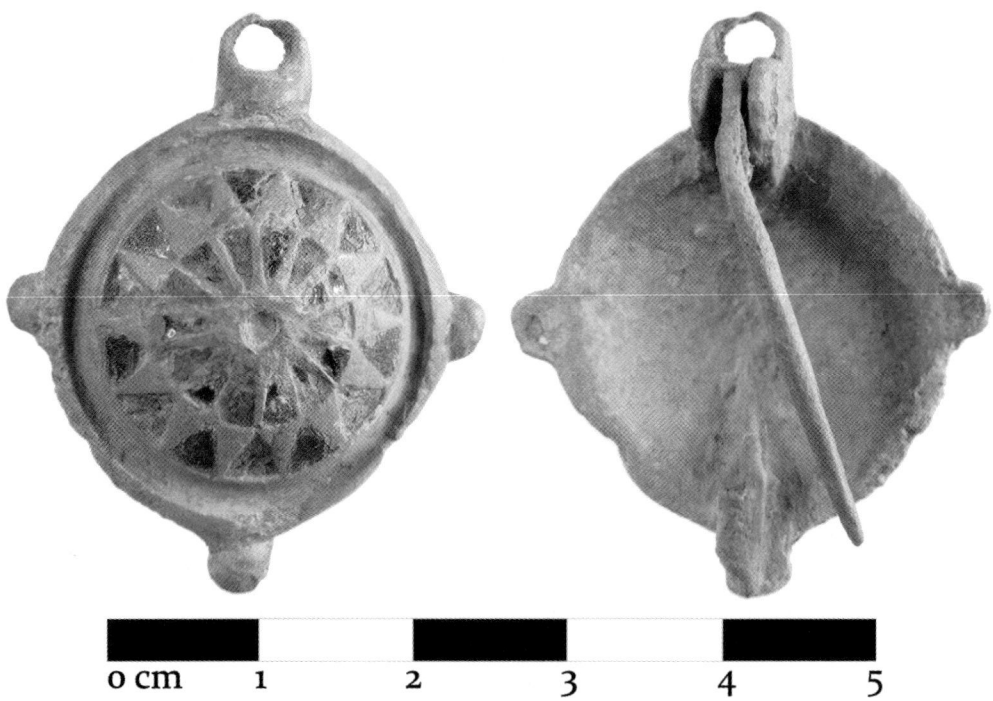

Fig. 4.4: Umbonate brooch with two rows of 14 cells for enamels found in Hampshire. PAS: HAMP-515B13 (PAS finds reproduced under Creative Commons Share-Alike Agreement).

brooch with applied silver decoration, from Wakefield, UK, PAS No. SWYOR-14EF37). If the richness of a brooch was understood, then the intent might be aspirational. Through the wearing of an object that was deliberately changed for it to appear luxurious, an owner may have wished to be associated with the elite, although in reality, it may have been the only 'luxurious' object the person owned.

Brooches for children

From an early age, people in the Roman north-west wore brooches, and they remained using them for the rest of their lives. Yet, not much attention in the literature has been devoted to the subject of brooch use by children, and this section is a short introduction into this issue.

The evidence suggests that brooches associated with children had roles that may have varied depending on their geographical location. In the Roman north-west they fulfilled their primary functional purpose of serving as pins. There is enough pictorial, textual and sculptural evidence to suggest that infant children were swaddled in bands wrapped around the entire infant's body until they reached 40–60 days old (Carroll 2012, 137–40; Derks 2014; Graham 2014). Babies between the ages of 4 or 6 months to 1 year were also swaddled but in a shroud that was most likely pinned at the shoulder. Bone pins were usually used, but sometimes also brooches (Carroll 2012, 140), evidenced by brooches found in infant children's graves. A brooch positioned near the shoulder of an infant three to four months old was found buried under the floor of a Roman pottery workshop at Sallèles D'Aude, southern France, where it was plausibly used to fix a shroud around the body of a child just as it was swaddled (Carroll 2012, 140 citing Duday 2009, 63–9). Further evidence for the use of brooches as pins to fasten a shroud in infant burials comes from beyond the Roman frontier. In a Roman Iron Age burial at Dunbar, Scotland, a penannular brooch was found near the rib area of 30–40 month old child (Hunter 2002, 210; 2013b, 276).

In the area covering the modern northern German state Mecklenburg-Vorpommern, brooches were frequently deposited in children's graves. Use-wear analysis on these locally produced brooches of the second century has shown that brooches with minimal or no signs of wear were predominantly deposited in the graves of children below the age of 10 (von Richthofen 1998, 254). The low intensity of wear indicates that these brooches had been used for a period of less than ten years before their deposition (von Richthofen 1998, 254). This could perhaps be seen as an indication of their use by these young children, who were buried with the personal objects they wore in life. Such evidence is yet to be found in the Roman north-west, but as adults living in Roman provinces pinned their cloaks with brooches, children may also have needed brooches to pin their clothes in the similar fashion. This is also suggested by pictorial evidence: tombstones commemorating boys aged three to fourteen show them depicted with their cloaks pinned to the right shoulder with disc brooches, in a similar manner to their fathers (Fig. 4.5; *cf.* also Lupa Nr. 1266, 2433, 3530, 4344, 4380, 4613, 5164, 12311, and 19743).

The question here is whether these disc brooches worn by children on sculptural reliefs were there to emphasise that they were from a well-to-do family, as was plausibly the case with the adults depicted in this manner (see above; also Lupa Nr. 3530 is an image of a four-year old male child whose father was a *beneficiarius tribuni*; Lupa Nr. 19743 is a portrait of a young Caracalla). The artistic representation of male children with these brooches may have been connected to the social articulation of notions of masculinity and social position rather than with childishness or youth. Depicting male children in what appears to be adult attire conspicuously fastened with the badge of masculinity and possibly adulthood may have been an intentional convention meant

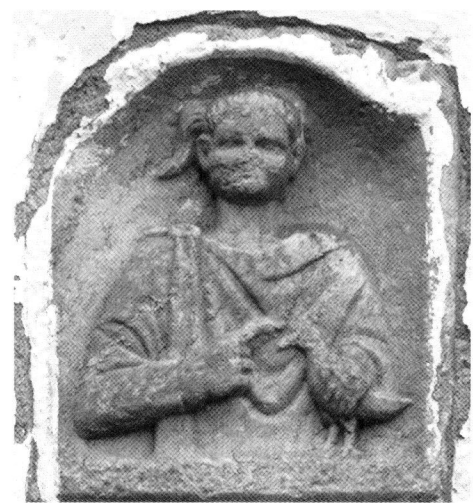

Fig. 4.5: Tombstone of a deceased 4-year old Vibius. Found in Hohenstein/Liebenfels, Austria. (Lupa 861-B1; ©Ortolf Harl 2003).

to convey an idealised conception of age, status and wealth (Carroll 2012, 144; 2014, 161–2, 172). These emblematic disc brooches on tombstones therefore made the male children into wealthy and powerful adults in perpetuity on the funerary stone reliefs. Brooches here fulfilled the role of status objects rather than of commodity or personal decorations.

In the burials of Mecklenburg-Vorpommern brooches were also valued as handled objects that may have connected the generations. Analysis suggested that heavily used brooches also appear in the graves of children below the age of ten, fulfilling, therefore, the role of heirlooms (von Richthofen 1998, 254). In this case, it is their physical properties of being old artefacts that made them favoured for children's burials. Due to their age they may have been seen as inter-generational objects protecting the remains of a child (paraphrasing Gilchrist 2013, 372 on the nature of medieval heirlooms as having '*spiritual* power that made them the equivalent of amulets or relics, sacred objects with quasi-magical properties of healing and *protection*' (my emphasis)). This role as inter-generational emotive objects is yet to be tested in relation to the brooches found within the borders of the Roman Empire.

Another problem that needs to be outlined here briefly is how to define children's brooches. Are they defined by size or imagery? In the above-mentioned example of the penannular brooch from the burial at Dunbar excavators have noticed its small size, tentatively calling it 'a specifically child-sized brooch' (Hunter 2002, 210). Similar examples were found all across Roman Iron Age Scotland but not in connection with child burials (Hunter 2002, 210). Children in the Roman north-west were sometimes depicted on their tombstones holding or touching animals, which, in the majority of the cases, were exclusively attributed to children (Mander 2013, 54). Brooches were also produced in the forms of many animals, such as horses, hares and rabbits, dogs, ducks and cockerels, among others. These zoomorphic plate brooches were rather small and incapable of holding thick and heavy adult cloaks. One may therefore suggest that zoomorphic brooches may have been used to decorate children's cloaks or acted as a third decorative ornament on their costume, alluding to children's toys. Yet, most research on zoomorphic brooches has convincingly shown that most types were badges or symbols signifying membership of particular religious cults and could be linked to the worship of particular deities (Allason-Jones 2014; Simpson and Blance 1998; *cf.* also Crummy 2007 on cockerel brooches; Johns 1995 on brooches in the forms of ducks and Fillery-Travis 2012 on horse-and-rider brooches). Wearers of such brooches were making visual statements related to their visits to deities' shrines (acting as pilgrim badges), their protection and personal beliefs, although one should not forget that such badges may not have necessarily been worn by adults.

Instead of a conclusion: what brooches do not do

The approach proposed here emphasises the active role of Roman brooches in human-object relationships and sees these mundane objects as the intelligent products of human action, being at the same time also containers and shapers of emotions, feelings and thoughts (after Gosden 2010, 40–1 on the house as an intelligent object). The importance of brooches in the Roman north-west, their multivocality and *Funktionswandel* have been shown, but this does not mean that brooches were the most important dress accessory. They were not the only items worn in the Roman Empire: belts (see Hoss, this volume), ear-rings, rings, bracelets, and hairpins constituted a person's dress practices, contesting his or her socially imposed identities and forming the canvas of the individual. One should also

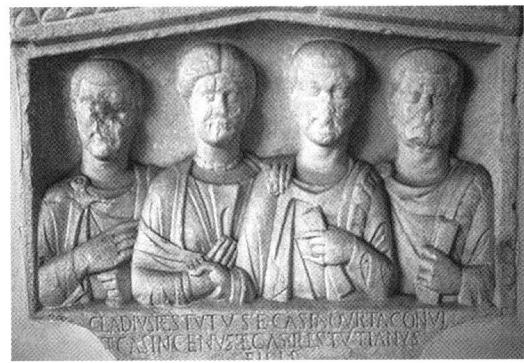

Fig. 4.6: *Tombstone depicting a family with three men wearing disc brooches. Found in Strass in Steiermark, Austria (Lupa 1355-1; ©Ortolf Harl).*

not forget that brooches were not the only objects to fasten clothes; metal and bone pins were commonly used. Figure 4.6 clearly shows that in some areas, for some dress types, women had no need for brooches (*cf.* also Allason-Jones 2013, 24: 'The inhabitants of Lepcis Magna had no need for brooches'). Furthermore, there was sometimes no need for men to wear them. *Paenulae* cloaks, popular in the second century AD, did not require brooches, as they were fastened with button-and-loop fasteners (Wild 1970). Thus, if a person did not wear brooches, it does not mean that he or she could not manifest themselves via other personal adornments (Allason-Jones 2013, 30).

This chapter should be seen as a first step towards establishing what brooches were at different times, their variety of functions, and also as an acknowledgement of their limitations. It is proposed to move beyond seeing brooches as identity markers only, since this is only one of multiple active functions carried out by brooches. Understanding the multi-functionality and plurality of a brooch in the Roman north-west in the first to third centuries AD will provide a more eclectic and nuanced vision of the visual world, perceptions of the self and others, and societal and individual choices coalescing and mingling in the excessively colourful Roman world.

Acknowledgments

This contribution was written during my fellowship in the TOPOI excellence cluster and Berliner Antike-Kolleg. While this piece is not a direct outcome of the project, my presence in Berlin on account of the fellowship and my participation in the theoretical discussions and workshops organised during my stay greatly contributed to the ideas developed in the text. I wish to thank the following people who consciously and unconsciously contributed to the ideas expressed in the text: Kerstin Hofmann, Stefan Schreiber, Arnica Kesseler, and Miguel-John Versluys. Special thanks are due to Rosie Weetch and Toby Martin for inviting me to contribute to this volume and their comments and suggestions for the improvement of this paper. I give special thanks to Lupa picture database of antique stone monuments and Ortolf Harl for their kind permission to reproduce the images. All mistakes remain my own.

Abbreviations
CIL = *Corpus Inscriptionum Latinarum*
LUPA = picture database of antique stone monuments (http://www.ubi-erat-lupa.org)
PAS = Portable Antiquities Scheme (http://finds.org.uk/)

Bibliography
Abdy R., Williams J. H. C. and Hill J. D. (2004) Church Minshull, Cheshire. *Treasure Annual Report 2004*, 174–5.
Allason-Jones, L. (1995) Sexing small finds. In P. Rush (ed.) *Theoretical Roman Archaeology: Second Conference Proceedings*, 22–32. Aldershot, Avebury.
Allason-Jones, L. (2005) *Women in Roman Britain*. York, Council for British Archaeology.
Allason-Jones, L. (2013) Missing people, missing brooches. In G. Grabherr, B. Kainrath and T. Schierl (eds.) *Relations Abroad: Brooches and Other Elements of Dress as Sources for Reconstructing Interregional Movement and Group Boundaries from the Punic Wars to the Decline of the Western Roman Empire. Proceedings of the International Conference from 27th–29th April 2011 in Innsbruck*, 24–32. Innsbruck, Innsbruck University Press.
Allason-Jones, L. (2014) Zoomorphic brooches: decoration or ideology? In S.-R. Marzel and G. D. Stiebel (eds.) *Dress and Ideology: Fashioning Identity from Antiquity to the Present*, 69–87. London: Bloomsbury.
Allison, P. (2013) *People and Spaces in Roman Military Bases*. Cambridge, Cambridge University Press.
Antonaccio, C. M. (2009) (Re)defining ethnicity: culture, material culture and identity. In S. Hales and T. Hodos (eds.) *Material Culture and Social Identities in the Ancient World*, 32–54. New York, Cambridge University Press.
Ball, J. (2014) Small finds and Roman battlefields: the process and impact of post-battle looting. In H. Platts, J. Pearce, C. Barron, J. Lundock and J. Yoo (eds.) *TRAC 2013. Proceedings of the Twenty-Third Theoretical Roman Archaeology Conference, King's College, London 2013*, 90–105. Oxford, Oxbow Books.
Bateson, J. D. and Hedges, R. E. M. (1975) The scientific analysis of a group of Roman-age enamelled brooches. *Archaeometry* 17(2), 177–90.
Bayley, J. and Butcher, S. (2004) *Roman Brooches in Britain: A Technological and Typological Study Base on the Richborough Collection*. London, Society of Antiquaries in London.
Booth, A. (2015) Reassessing the Long Chronology of the Penannular Brooch in Britain: Exploring Changing Styles, Use and Meaning Across a Millennium. Unpublished PhD thesis, University of Leicester.
Brather, S. (2004) *Ethnische Interpretationen in der frühgeschichtlichen Archäologie: Geschichte, Grundlage und Alternativen*. Berlin, De Gruyter.
Brather, S. (2009) Ethnische Identitäten aus archäologischer Perspektive. In *Kelten am Rhein. Akten des dreizehnten Internationalen Keltologiekongresses, 23. bis 27. Juli 2007 on Bonn. Vol. 1 Ethnizität und Romanisierung*, 1–12. Mainz, Philipp von Zabern.
Brubaker, R. and Cooper, F. (2000) Beyond "identity". *Theory and Society* 29, 1–47.
Böhme-Schönberger, A. (1994) Die Kragenfibel – eine treverische Fibelform? In C. Dobiat (ed.) *Festschrift für Otto-Herman Frey zum 65. Geburtstag*, 111–26. Marburg, Hitzeroth.
Böhme-Schönberger, A. (2002) Die Distelfibel und die Germanen. In K. Kuzmová, K. Pieta, J. Rajtár (eds.) *Zwischen Rom und dem Barbaricum. Festschrift für Titus Kolnik zum 70. Geburtstag*, 215–24. Nitra, Archäologisches Institut der Slowakischen Akademie der Wissenschaften.

Böhme-Schönberger, A. (2008) Die Distelfibeln – Sind sie Männer- oder Frauenfibeln? In U. Brandl (ed.) *Frauen und Römisches Militär: Beiträge eines Runden Tisches in Xanten vom 7. bis 9. Juli 2005*, 140–45. Oxford, Archaeopress (British Archaeological Reports, International Series 1759).

Butcher, S. (1977) Enamels from Roman Britain. In M. R. Apted, R., Gilyard-Beer, A. D. Saunders, and A. J. Taylor (eds.) *Ancient Monuments and their Interpretation: Essays Presented to A. J. Taylor*, 41–69. London, Phillimore.

Butcher, S. (1986) The brooches. In R. Leech (ed.) The excavation of a Romano-Celtic temple and a later cemetery on Lamyatt Beacon, Somerset. *Britannia* 17, 259–328.

Butler, J. (1993) *Bodies that matter: On the Discursive Limits of Sex*. London, Routledge.

Callewaert, M. (2012) Les fibules romaines : archéologie, usages et fonctions. In P. Cattelain, N. Bozet and G. V. Di Stazio (eds.) *La parure de Cro-Magnon à Clovis: "Il n'y a pas d'Âge(s) pour se Faire Beau"*, 117–34. Treignes, Centre d'études et de recherche archéologiques (Cedarc).

Canny, D. and Dilly, G. (1997) Les fibules de Fesques. In E. Mantel (ed.) *Le sanctuaire de Fesques: "Le mont du Val aux Moines" (Seine Maritime)*, 185–99. Berck sur Mer, CRADC.

Carroll, M. (2012) The Roman child clothed in death. In M. Carroll and J. P. Wild (eds.) *Dressing the Dead in Classical Antiquity*, 134–48. Stroud, Amberley.

Carroll, M. (2014) Mother and infant in Roman funerary commemoration. In M. Carroll and E.-J. Graham (eds.) *Infant Health and Death in Roman Italy and Beyond*, 159–79. Portsmouth, RI, Journal of Roman Archaeology.

Casella, E. C., Fowler, C., eds. (2005) *The Archaeology of Plural and Changing Identities: Beyond Identification*. New York, Kluwer Academic/Plenum Publishers.

Cool, H. E. M. (1983) A Study of the Roman Personal Ornaments Made of Metal. Unpublished PhD thesis, University of Wales.

Collins, R. (2010) Brooch use in the frontier from the 4th–5th centuries. In R. Collins and L. Allason-Jones (eds.) *Finds from the Frontier: Material Culture in the 4th-5th Centuries*, 64–77. York, Council for British Archaeology (Council for British Archaeology Research Report 162).

Croom, A. (2002) *Roman Clothing and Fashion*. Stroud, Tempus.

Crummy, N. (2007) Brooches and the cult of Mercury. *Britannia* 38, 225–30.

Curta, F. (2005) Female dress and "Slavic" bow *fibulae* in Greece. *Hesperia* 74(1), 101–46.

Derks, T. (2009) Ethnic identity in the Roman frontier. The epigraphy of Batavi and other Lower Rhine tribes. In T. Derks and N. Roymans (eds.), *Ethnic Constructs in Antiquity: The Role of Power and Tradition*, 239–283. Amsterdam, Amsterdam University Press.

Derks, T. (2014) Protection against ultimately death: infant votives from Gaul and Germany. In M. Carroll and E.-J. Graham (eds.) *Infant Health and Death in Roman Italy and Beyond*, 47–69. Portsmouth, RI, Journal of Roman Archaeology.

Devillers, S. (2000) Les fibules du sanctuaire de la forêt d'Halatte (commune d'Ognon, Oise). *Revue archéologique de Picardie* 18, 267–76.

Diaz-Andreu, M. (2005) Gender identity. In M. Diaz-Andreu and S. Lucy (eds.) *Archaeology of Identities: Approaches to Gender, Age, Status, Ethnicity and Religion*, 13–42. London, Routledge.

Diaz-Andreu, M. and Lucy, S. (2005) Introduction. In M. Diaz-Andreu and S. Lucy (eds.) *Archaeology of Identities: Approaches to Gender, Age, Status, Ethnicity and Religion*, 1–12. London, Routledge.

Dollfus, J. (1973) *Catalogue des Fibules de Bronze de Haute-Normandie*. Paris, Imprimerie Nationale.

Duday, H. (2009) *The Archaeology of the Dead. Lectures in Archaeothanalogy*. Oxford, Oxbow Books.

Eckardt, H. (2005) The social distribution of Roman artefacts: the case of nail cleaners and brooches in Britain. *Journal of Roman Archaeology* 18, 139–60.

Eckardt, H. (2014) *Objects and Identities. Roman Britain and the North-Western Provinces*. Oxford, Oxford University Press.

Edgar, M. (2012) Beyond Typology: Late Iron Age and Early Roman Brooches in Northern France. Unpublished PhD thesis, University of Leicester.

Faider-Feytmans, G. (1965) *La Nécropole Gallo-Romaine de Thuin*. Morlanwelz, Musée de Mariemont.

Fauduet, I. and C. Pommeret (1985) Les fibules du sanctuaire des Bolards à Nuits-Saint-George (Côte d'or). *Revue Archéologique de L'Est et du Centre-Est* 36, 63–116.

Feugère, M. (1985) *Les Fibules en Gaule Méridionale, de la Conquête à la Fin du 7e s. apr. J.-C.* Paris, Centre National de la Recherche Scientifique.

Fibel und Fibeltracht (2011). 2. Auflage. Berlin/Boston, De Gruyter.

Fillery-Travis, R. (2012) Multidisciplinary analysis of Roman horse-and-rider brooches from Bosworth. In I. Schrüfer-Kolb (ed.) *More Than Just Numbers? The Role of Science in Roman Archaeology*, 135–63. Portsmouth, RI, Journal of Roman Archaeology.

Flowers, H. (2011) Adorning identities: brooches as social strategy in Early Medieval Europe. In L. Amundsen-Meyer, N. Engel and S. Pickering (eds.) *Identity Crisis: Archaeological Perspectives on Social Identity*, 27–36. Calgary, Chacmool Archaeological Association.

Fowler, C. (2004) *The Archaeology of Personhood: An Anthropological Approach.* London, Routledge.

Garbsch, J, (1965) *Die norisch-pannonische Frauentracht im 1. und 2. Jahrhundert.* Munich, Beck.

Gardner, A. (2007) *An Archaeology of Identity: Soldiers and Society in Late Roman Britain.* Walnut Creek, Left Coast Press.

Gardner, A. (2013) Thinking about Roman imperialism: postcolonialism, globalisation and beyond? *Britannia* 44, 1–25.

Gell, A. (1998) *Art and Agency: An Anthropological Theory.* Oxford, Clarendon Press.

Gilchrist, R. (2013) The materiality of medieval heirlooms: from biographical to sacred objects. In H. P. Hahn and H. Weiss (eds.) *Mobility, Meaning and Transformation of Things: Shifting Contexts of Material Culture through Time and Space*, 170–83. Oxford, Oxbow Books.

Gosden, C. (2010) The death of the mind. In L. Malafouris and C. Renfew (eds.) *The Cognitive Life of Things: Recasting the Boundaries of the Mind*, 39–46. Cambridge, McDonald Institute Monographs.

Grabherr, G., Kainrath, B., and Schierl, T., eds. (2013) *Relations Abroad: Brooches and Other Elements of Dress as Sources for Reconstructing Interregional Movement and Group Boundaries from the Punic Wars to the Decline of the Western Roman Empire. Proceedings of the International Conference from 27th-29th April 2011 in Innsbruck.* Innsbruck, Innsbruck University Press.

Graham, E.-J. (2014) Infant votives and swaddling in Hellenistic Italy. In M. Carroll and E.-J. Graham (eds.) *Infant Health and Death in Roman Italy and Beyond*, 23–46. Portsmouth, RI, Journal of Roman Archaeology.

Grane, T. (2013) Roman imports in Scandinavia: their purpose and meaning? In P. Wells (ed.) *Rome Beyond its Frontiers: Imports, Attitudes and Practices*, 29–44. Portsmouth, RI, Journal of Roman Archaeology.

Guillaumet, J.-P. (1984) *Les Fibules de Bibracte. Technique et Typologie.* Dijon, Université de Dijon.

Hahn, H. P. and Weiss, H., eds. (2013) *Mobility, Meaning and Transformation of Things: Shifting Contexts of Material Culture through Time and Space.* Oxford, Oxbow Books.

Harlow, M. ed. (2012) *Dress and Identity.* Oxford, Archaeopress (British Archaeological Reports, International Series 2356).

Harrison, G. (1999) Quoit brooches and the Roman-Medieval transition. In P. Baker, C. Forcey, S. Jundi and R. Witcher (eds.) *TRAC 98: Proceedings of the Eighth Annual Theoretical Roman Archaeology Conference Leicester 1998.* 108–20. Oxford, Oxbow Books.

Heeren, S. (2014) Brooches and burials: variability in expressions of identity in cemeteries of the Batavian *civitas*. *Journal of Roman Archaeology* 27, 443–55.

Heynowski, R. (2012) *Fibeln: Erkennen, Bestimmen, Beschreiben.* Altenburg, Deutscher Kunstverlag.

Hingley, R. (2005) *Globalazing Roman Culture: Unity, Diversity and Empire.* London, Routledge.

Hodder, I. (2011). Human–thing entanglement: towards an integrated archaeological perspective. *Journal of the Royal Anthropological Institute* 17, 154–77.

Hodder, I. (2012) *Entangled: An Archaeology of the Relationships Between Humans and Things.* Oxford, Wiley-Blackwell.

Hodos, T. (2010) Local and global perspectives in the study of social and cultural identities. In S. Hales and T. Hodos (eds.) *Material Culture and Social Identities in the Ancient World*, 3–31. New York, Cambridge University Press.

Hofmann, K. P. and Schreiber, T. (2011) Mit Lanzetten durch den *practical turn*. Zum Wechselspiel zwischen Mensch und Ding aus archäologischer Perspektive. *EAZ-Ethnographisch-Archäologische Zeitschrift* 52(2), 163–87.

Hunter, F. (2002) The penannular brooch. In L. Baker, (ed.) An Iron Age child burial at Dunbar Golf Course, East Lothian. *Proceedings of the Society of Antiquaries of Scotland* 132, 205–12.

Hunter, F. (2008) Celtic art in Roman Britain. In D. Garrow, C. Gosden and J. D. Hill (eds.) *Rethinking Celtic Art*, 129–45. Oxford, Oxbow Books.

Hunter, F. (2010) Changing objects in changing worlds: dragonesque brooches and beaded torcs. In S. Worrell, G. Egan, J. Naylor, *et al.* (eds.) *A Decade of Discovery: Proceedings of the Portable Antiquities Scheme Conference 2007*, 91–107. Oxford, Archaeopress (British Archaeological Reports, British Series 520).

Hunter, F. (2013a) The lives of Roman objects beyond the frontier. In P. Wells (ed.) *Rome Beyond its Frontiers: Imports, Attitudes and Practices*, 15–28. Portsmouth, RI, Journal of Roman Archaeology.

Hunter, F. (2013b) Roman brooches around and across the British *limes*. In G. Grabherr, B. Kainrath and T. Schierl (eds.) *Relations Abroad: Brooches and Other Elements of Dress as Sources for Reconstructing Interregional Movement and Group Boundaries from the Punic Wars to the Decline of the Western Roman Empire. Proceedings of the International Conference from 27th–29th April 2011 in Innsbruck*, 270–280. Innsbruck, Innsbruck University Press.

Ingold, T. (2007) Materials against materiality. *Archaeological Dialogues*, 14(1), 1–16.

Insoll, T. (2007) Introduction. Configuring identities in archaeology. In T. Insoll (ed.), *The Archaeology of Identities: A Reader*, 1–18. London, Routledge.

Ivleva, T. (2011) British emigrants in the Roman Empire: complexities and symbols of ethnic identities. In D. Mladenovič and B. Russell (eds.), *TRAC 2010: Proceedings of the Twentieth Annual Theoretical Roman Archaeology Conference, Oxford 2010*, 132–53. Oxford, Oxbow Books.

Ivleva, T. (2012) Britons Abroad: The Mobility of Britons and the Circulation of British-Made Objects in the Roman Empire. Unpublished PhD thesis, University of Leiden.

Ivleva, T. (2016) A totality of a thing with objects: multifaceted British-made brooches abroad. In K. P. Hofmann, T. Meier, D. Mölders, and St Schreiber (eds.) *Massendinghaltung in der Archäologie. Der material turn und die Ur- und Frühgeschichte*, 365–86. Leiden, Sidestone Press.

Johns, C. (1995) Mounted men and sitting ducks: the iconography of Romano-British plate-brooches. In B. Raftery, V. Megaw and V. Rigby (eds.) *Sites and Sights of the Iron Age: Essays on Fieldwork and Museum Research Presented to Ian Mathieson*, 105–109. Oxford Oxbow Books.

Johns, C. (1996) *The Jewellery of Roman Britain: Celtic and Classical Traditions*. London, University of College London Press.

Johns, C. (2002) Romeinse schatvondsten in Noordwest-Europa. In K. Sas and H. Thoen (eds.), *Schone Schijn. Romeinse juweelkunst in West-Europa*, 71–83. Leuven, Peeters.

Jones, S. (1997) *The Archaeology of Ethnicity: Constructing Identities in the Past and Present*. London, Routledge.

Jundi, S. and Hill, J. D. (1998) Brooches and identities in first century AD Britain: more than meets the eye? In C. Forcey, J. Hawthrone and R. Witcher (eds.) *TRAC 97: Proceedings of the Seventh Annual Theoretical Roman Archaeology Conference, Nottingham 1997*, 125–37. Oxford, Oxbow Books.

Kopytoff, I. (1986) Cultural biography of things: commoditization as process. In A. Appadurai (ed.) *The Social Life of Things: Commodities in Cultural Perspective*, 64–91. Cambridge, Cambridge University Press.

Laet, de, S. J., van Doorselaer, A., Spitaels, P. and Thoen, H. (1972) *La Nécropole Gallo-Romaine de Blicquy (Hainaut-Belgique)*. Brugge, De Temple.

Láng, M. (1919) Die pannonische Frauentracht. *Jahreshefte des Österreichischen Archäologischen Institutes in Wien*, 19–20, 207–60.

Latour, B. (2005) *Reassembling the Social: An Introduction to Actor-Network-Theory*. Oxford, Oxford University Press.

Leifeld, H. (2007) *Endlatène- und älterkaiserzeitliche Fibeln aus Gräbern des Trierer Landes: Eine antiquarisch-chronologische Studie*. Bonn, Rudolf Habelt.

Lucy, S. (2005) Ethnic and cultural identities. In M. Diaz-Andreu and S. Lucy (eds.) *The Archaeology of Identity: Approaches to Gender, Age, Status, Ethnicity and Religion*, 86–109. London, Routledge.

Mackreth, D. F. (2011) *Brooches in Late Iron Age and Roman Britain*. Oxford, Oxbow Books.

Malafouris, L., Renfew, C. (2010) Introduction. The cognitive life of things: archaeology, material engagement and the extended mind. In L. Malafouris and C. Renfew (eds.) *The Cognitive Life of Things: Recasting the Boundaries of the Mind*, 1–12. Cambridge, McDonald Institute Monographs.

Mander, J. (2013) *Portraits of Children on Roman Funerary Monuments*. Cambridge, Cambridge University Press.

Mattingly, D. (2004) Being Roman: expressing identity in a provincial setting. *Journal of Roman Archaeology* 17, 5–25.

Mattingly, D. (2011) *Imperialism, Power, and Identity: Experiencing the Roman Empire*. Princeton, Princeton University Press.

McIntosh, F. (2010) The Wirral Brooch: the Form, Distribution and Role of a Romano-British Type. Unpublished MLitt Thesis, University of Newcastle upon Tyne.

McIntosh, F. (2011) Regional brooch-types in Roman Britain: evidence from northern England. *Archaeologia Aeliana* (fifth series) 40, 155–82.

McIntosh, F. (2013) The Wirral brooch – a rural and regional brooch type. In G. Grabherr, B. Kainrath and T. Schierl (eds.) *Relations Abroad: Brooches and Other Elements of Dress as Sources for Reconstructing Interregional Movement and Group Boundaries from the Punic Wars to the Decline of the Western Roman Empire. Proceedings of the International Conference from 27th-29th April 2011 in Innsbruck*, 257–69. Innsbruck, Innsbruck University Press.

Meskell, L. (2007) Archaeologies of identity. In T. Insoll (ed.) *The Archaeology of Identities: A Reader*, 23–43. London, Routledge.

Olsen, B. (2010) *In Defense of Things: Archaeology and the Ontology of Objects*. Lanham MD, AltaMira Press.

Parker Pearson, M. (1999) *The Archaeology of Death and Burial*. Stroud, Sutton.

Pearce, J. (2011) Representations and realities: cemeteries as evidence for women in Roman Britain. *Medicina nei Secoli Arte e Scienza* 23(1), 227–54.

Philippe, J. (1999) *Les Fibules de Seine-et-Marne du 1er Siècle av. J.-C. au 5e Siècle ap. J.-C.* Nemours, Service départemental d'Archéologie de Seine-et-Marne.

Philpott, R. (1991) *Burial Practices in Roman Britain: A Survey of Grave Treatment and Furnishing, A.D. 43-410*. Oxford, Tempus Reparatum (British Archaeological Reports, British Series 219).

Philpott, R. A. (1993) Personal ornament and burial practices in Roman Britain. In M. Struck (ed.) *Römerzeitliche Gräber als Quellen zu Religion, Bevölkerungsstruktur und Sozialgeschichte*, 167–179. Mainz, Institut für Vor- und Frühgeschichte der Johannes-Gutenberg-Universität Mainz.

Pitts, M. (2007) The Emperor's new clothes? The utility of identity in Roman archaeology. *American Journal of Archaeology* 111, 693–713.

Pohl, W. (1998) Telling the difference: signs of ethnic identity. In W. Pohl (ed.) *Strategies of Distinction: The Construction of Ethnic Communities, 300-800*, 17–94. Leiden, Brill.

Pollock, K. J. (2006) *The Evolution and Role of Burial Practice in Roman Wales*. Oxford, John and Erica Hedges (British Archaeological Reports, British Series 426).

Pudney, C. (2011) Pinning down identity: the negotiation of personhood and the materialisation of identity in the Late Iron Age and Early Roman Severn estuary. In D. Mladenović and B. Russell (eds.), *TRAC 2010: Proceedings of the Twentieth Annual Theoretical Roman Archaeology Conference, Oxford 2010*, 115–31. Oxford, Oxbow Books.

Pulles, I. and Roymans, N. (1994) Mantelspelden en armringen als offerobject. In N. Roymans, and T. Derks (eds.) *De Tempel van Empel. Een Hercules-heiligdom in het Woongebied van de Bataven*, 132–41. 's Hertogenbosch, Stichting Brabantse Regionale Geschiedbeoefening.

Revell, L. (2009) *Roman Imperialism and Local Identities*. Cambridge, Cambridge University Press.

Richthofen, von, J. (1998) Gebrauchsspuren an Fibeln der älteren römischen Kaiserzeit und Ergebnisse der Materialprüfung. *Bericht der Römisch-Germanischen Kommission* 79, 242–59.

Rothe, U. (2012a) Dress and cultural identity in the Roman Empire. In M. Harlow (ed.) *Dress and Identity*, 59–69. Oxford, Archaeopress (British Archaeological Reports, International Series 2356).

Rothe, U. (2012b) The "Third Way": Treveran women's dress and the "Gallic Ensemble". *American Journal of Archaeology* 116, 235–52.

Rothe, U. (2013) Die norisch-pannonische Tracht – gab es sie wirklich? In G. Grabherr, B. Kainrath and T. Schierl (eds) *Relations Abroad: Brooches and Other Elements of Dress as Sources for Reconstructing Interregional Movement and Group Boundaries from the Punic Wars to the Decline of the Western Roman Empire. Proceedings of the International Conference from 27th–29th April 2011 in Innsbruck*, 34–48. Innsbruck, Innsbruck University Press.

Rowlands, M. (2007) The politics of identity in archaeology. In T. Insoll (ed.) *The Archaeology of Identities: a Reader*, 59–71. London, Routledge.

Schörner, G., ed. (2005) *Romanisierung-Romanisation: theoretische Modelle und praktische Fallbeispiele*. Oxford, Archaeopress (British Archaeological Reports, International Series 1427).

Simpson, G. and Blance, B. (1998) Do brooches have ritual associations? In J. Bird (ed.) *Form and Fabric: Studies in Rome's Material Past in Honour of B. R. Hartley*, 267–81. Oxford Oxbow Books.

Snape, M. (1993) *Roman Brooches from North Britain: A Classification and a Catalogue of Brooches from Sites on the Stanegate*. Oxford, Tempus Reparatum (British Archaeological Reports, British Series 235).

Swift, E. (2000) *Regionality in Dress Accessories in the Late Roman West*. Montagnac, Monique Mergoil.

Swift, E. (2003) Transformations in meaning: amber and glass beads across the Roman frontier. In G. Carr, E. Swift and J. Weeks (eds.) *TRAC 2002: Proceedings of the Twelfth Annual Theoretical Roman Archaeology Conference, Canterbury 2002*, 48–57. Oxford, Oxbow Books.

Tilley, C. (2004) *The Materiality of Stone: Explorations in Landscape Phenomenology*. Oxford, Berg.

Turkle, S. (2007) What makes an object evocative? In S. Turkle (ed.) *Evocative Objects: Things We Think with*, 307–28. Cambridge, MA, The MIT press.

Van Impe, L., and Creemers, G. (2002) Erfstukken uit een Keltische juwelenkist. In K. Sas and H. Thoen (eds.), *Schone Schijn. Romeinse juweelkunst in West-Europa*, 43–53. Leuven, Peeters.

Versluys, M.-J. (2014) Understanding objects in motion. An *archaeological* dialogue on Romanisation. *Archaeological Dialogues* 21(1), 1–20.

Versluys, M.-J. (2017) Egypt as part of the Roman koine: a study in mnemohistory. In S. Nagel, J. F. Quack and C. Witschel (eds.), *Entangled Worlds: Religious Confluences between East and West in the Roman Empire*. Tuebingen, Mohr Siebeck.

Vodoz, V. (1983) Les fibules du sanctuaire indigène de Martigny. *Archäologie der Schweiz* 2, 78–81.

Völling, T. (1994) Studien zu Fibelformen der jüngeren vorrömischen Eisenzeit und ältesten römischen Kaiserzeit. *Bericht der Römisch-Germanischen Kommission* 75, 147–282.

Wallace-Hadrill, A. (2007) The creation and expression of identity: the Roman world. In S. Alcock and R. Osborne (eds.) *Classical Archaeology*, 355–380. Oxford, Blackwell.

Wild, J. P. (1970) Button-and-loop fasteners in the Roman provinces. *Britannia* 1, 137–55.

Chapter 5

The Roman military belt – a status symbol and object of fashion

Stefanie Hoss

Introduction

The Roman military belt (called a *balteus* in the first century AD and a *cingulum militare* from the third century AD onwards, see Hoss 2011, 30), a leather belt closed with a buckle and decorated with metal mounts and hangers, was part of the military equipment of the Roman soldier and was worn both during battle and as a part of everyday dress. The military belts worn by the Late Roman army and their Barbaric *foederati* and successors during the transition from Late Antiquity to the Early Middle Ages (fourth to eighth centuries AD) have long been known as iconic items of dress, identifying their wearers as soldiers/warriors and almost overloaded with symbolism. They are central to the archaeological record of the period, and several major studies have investigated them (Bullinger 1969; Böhme 1974; Sommer 1984; Swift 2000). Although many researchers have recognised the importance of the Late Roman military belt, the question of how, when and why the belt attained such importance has only lately been the subject of further study. This is especially surprising considering the quantity and quality of the surviving evidence (see below).

In addition to these main issues, other research questions revolve around the decoration of the belt mounts – were they commissioned by a central authority or was it a matter of free choice for the soldiers? If the latter, what was the mechanism that enabled the apparently simultaneous changes from one design to the next? And what was pictured on this belt? Did the depictions resemble those on the armour and helmets of the soldiers or were they independent of them? Were the decorations characteristic for a certain unit or were they used in wider groups such as the armies on the Rhine or Danube or even the whole Roman army? These and many more technical questions were the starting points for my investigation into the Roman military belt (Hoss in prep.).

5. The Roman military belt – a status symbol and object of fashion

Evidence for military belts is made up of three categories. The first is a fairly small number of written sources, mainly papyri and the works of ancient authors (see Hoss 2013). The second category consists of more than 300 depictions on reliefs portraying Roman soldiers, either official triumphal monuments or the tombstones of the soldiers themselves. The latter are especially informative, as the soldiers here present themselves for posterity wearing their military belt, but only some of their arms and armour (Figs. 5.1 and 5.4, for a discussion of these monuments see Hoss 2011, 31–4). The reason for this choice of dress was to ensure that they were visually recognisable as individuals and as soldiers. Depiction in full armour with a helmet with closed cheek-pieces would have made recognition of the face impossible. But the visual representation of their chosen profession must also have been very important, because most tombstones in their inscriptions explicitly mention the service of the deceased and the most important posts they held – so a depiction was not strictly necessary to convey the deceased's profession.

The third and largest source of evidence is comprised of thousands of archaeological finds. As the leather has usually perished, it is the metal belt buckles, mounts and hangers that

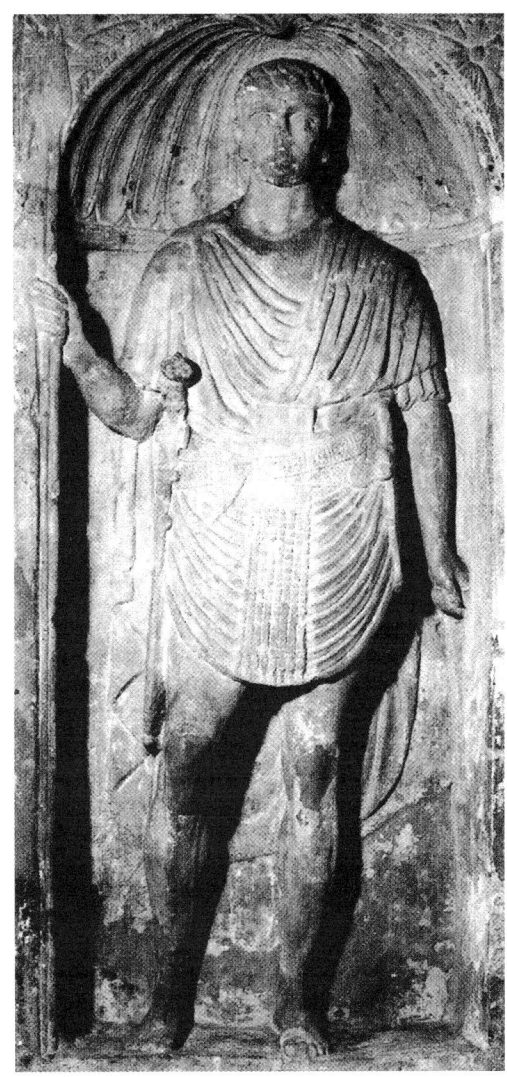

Fig. 5.1: Funerary monument of the soldier Publius Flavoleuis Cordus from Klein-Winternheim (near Mainz/D), dated between 15 and 43 AD (after Miks 2007, pl. 306C).

make up our picture of the military belt. Found in excavations in the Roman Empire (and in some instances outside of it), most finds of metal belt pieces were made individually, the pieces having been lost or broken and either thrown away or put aside for recycling in antiquity. Only finds from graves or rare catastrophic events (like the Vesuvius eruption) have preserved all the metal decorations of a single military belt in more or less the right order. Due to the funeral ritual observed at the time, weapons and equipment are exceptional grave goods during the first century

(Fischer 2011, 89). This seems to change during the course of the second and third centuries AD and finds of metal belt elements in graves become more common, but complete sets of belt mounts are still rare. The distribution of the finds over the Roman Empire is uneven, but this is a consequence of the fact that excavation and publication of archaeological sites is common in North-western Europe, less so in South-eastern Europe and rather an exception in North Africa and the Levant. The finds known from the few published excavations in the latter (Dura Europos in Syria, for instance) demonstrate that similar belt mounts were in use at roughly the same time over the whole Empire.

While most metal belt pieces have been found in excavations of auxiliary forts and legionary fortresses, examples from the civilian settlements, refuse dumps and cemeteries surrounding those military installations are common as well. Finds without a direct military connection are rarer, but by no means unusual, as Roman soldiers often travelled far and wide through the Empire, accompanying officials, procuring food and equipment for their unit or visiting their family.

During the three centuries under investigation, the belt changed considerably in appearance. In the first century AD, the Roman military belt consisted of one or two leather straps (serving as a 'foundation' for the belt), with widths of about 4–5cm, from which the sword hung on the right side and the dagger on the left (Fig. 5.1). The leather straps were each decorated with a series of copper-alloy mounts of similar size, covering the whole front of the belt. These mounts had little practical use, but they might have stiffened the belt and prevented it from rolling up lengthwise. On the front, the so-called apron was fixed to the inside of the belt. It consisted of several leather straps carrying both copper-alloy mounts and free-swinging hangers. This 'apron' was completely without technical or practical function in protecting the soldier; in fact, it may even have been a hindrance, for experimental archaeology has shown that during rapid movement, such as running, the weighted straps swinging between the wearer's legs were prone to strike the wearer in the genitals (Bishop and Coulston 2006, 110). It does, however, seem to have an important function in making the status of the wearer both visible and audible (see below).

A complete change in the manner of wearing the belt took place during the Antonine period (138–161 AD). The suspension of the sword changed from the waist-belt to the shoulder-belt and the 'apron' was no longer worn. In addition, the whole 'design' of the belt changed from solid, silvered and decorated metal plates covering the belt leather to a design playing with the effect of gold-like bronze openwork plates with the leather visible through them, with some examples also decorated with colourful enamel (see Fig. 5.3a–e). In another complete fashion change in the third century, the fairly wide belt was closed with a ring-buckle, consisting of a simple ring, worn at the area of the belly button (see Fig. 5.3f and Fig. 5.4). The leather strap of the belt was passed through the ring from the back on both sides and back along the front. The strap was fixed by sliding mushroom-shaped studs fixed to the front of the belt through slits in the leather strap. While the strap was often fairly short on the wearer's left side, the strap was longer on the right side. It was usually brought back in a long crescent loop to the belt and tucked behind it. The strap was often split into two and always decorated with free-swinging hangers, dangling around the area of the knee. Some of these were suspended from the leather strap end, while others were partly mounted against the leather and were connected with a hinge to a free-swinging part. On some third-century depictions, the soldiers hold this end in their right hand and seem to play with it; thus directing the viewer's attention to the belt as a distinctive piece of equipment (see Fig. 5.4).

Identity, community and dress

As the social sciences have demonstrated, individual identity is characterised by a complex and fluid matrix of different positions in a number of social connections (Collins 2008, 47). The different positions of a single individual can be simultaneous and interacting, making it difficult to define them archaeologically. In contrast, group or communal identity, and especially differences between communities are easier to understand through archaeological research. Communities can be defined as social formations between families and tribes in size, existing within larger political or social bodies and are 'not [...] exclusively institutional' (Collins 2008, 48). The distinct features and characteristics of different types of community, especially in the realm of the physical experience of objects, provide archaeology with the tools to distinguish and describe what is often termed 'group identities' by archaeologists (Collins 2008, 48–9). The individual's grade of identification with a social community is dependent on many factors, such as shared beliefs and important characteristics. Long-time association is also important as the connection must be continuously negotiated and reinforced in order to remain relevant for the individual (Anderson 2009, 27–8).

Social communities develop through interaction with and dissociation from other communities (Hogg *et al.* 1995). The contrast between conspicuous (often external) features of the individual's own community, the so-called *ingroup*, as compared with other relevant group(s), the so-called *outgroup(s)*, is used to define the community (Sommer 2012, 259). These features often symbolise important values of the community.

The expression of communal identity in dress was recognised early in anthropological and archaeological research (Reinhard 2006, 115; Peoples and Bailey 2010, 260). Because of its high immediacy through its direct connection with the individual, personal appearances – running the whole gamut of dress, jewellery, accessories (hats, bags, etc.) and body modifications (haircuts, piercings, tattoos) – dress plays an important role in the definition and construction of identity. With the help of these modifications, individuals change their biological body into a socially relevant manifestation, creating and visualising their identity for others and for themselves (Sommer 2012, 257).

The manner in which these outer features are used to visualise individual identity is often compared to a code or language, with which the individual communicates

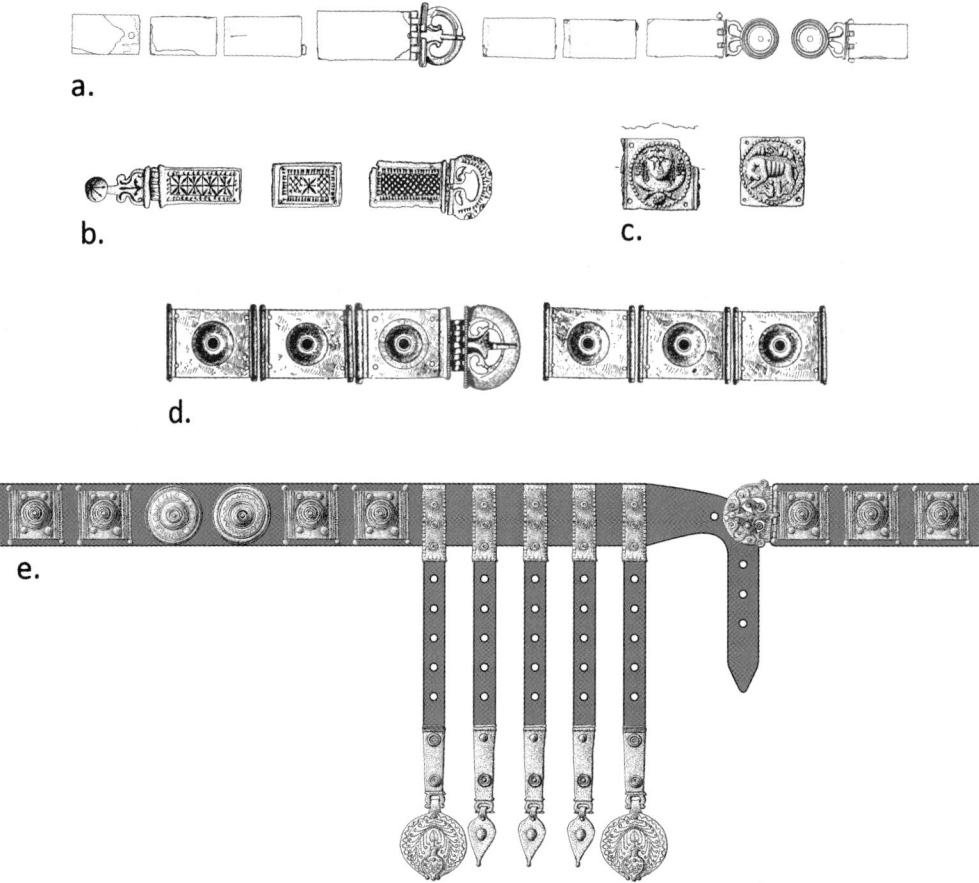

Fig. 5.2: Belt-sets, various dates: a. Velsen, first century (after Morel et al. 1989, fig. 5, 6); b. Hod Hill, first century AD (after Bishop and Coulston 2006, fig. 62); c. Risstissen and Oberstimm, first century AD (after Bishop and Coulston 2006, fig. 62); d. from the Rhine between Altrip and Rheingönheim, first century AD (after Ulbert 1969, pl. 32, 5); e. reconstruction of a Flavian belt, after the Tekije find (drawing A. Smadi, after Fischer 2012, fig. 111b).

his or her figurative position within society. The symbolic code of dress or clothing is highly ambivalent, and intimately connected with the (sub)society and period of its use (Sommer 2012, 257–8). In this code, the different signals are variations of the materials, cuts and colours used. The connotations connected to these in a given society are for the most part *conventionally arbitrary*, meaning, that they are the result of a socio-cultural agreement: not all societies view skirts as female dress or black as a mourning colour (Sommer 2012, 258).

Nevertheless, two key aspects in the 'code of dress' of most societies are (a) the social value given to the materials an item of dress is made of and (b) the way an item of dress will determine the body postures of its wearer (Sommer 2012, 257). While the fact that objects made from materials with a high (social) value tend to have a high value themselves is self-evident, the way dress determines body posture is less so. Items of dress can be used to encourage or restrict certain body movements; they can also enhance or hide certain parts of the body. The body postures encouraged in this manner are related to the social position of the wearer, and emphasise certain aspects seen as being an ideal for this position in that culture. While high heeled shoes or tight skirts result in the wearer being only able to take small and less than steady steps, this restriction of body movement has expressed an ideal for a young attractive female in numerous societies. Items of clothing promoting a straight back and enhancing the shoulders are often used for males. Such a body posture, whose main aim it is to make the individual seem larger, is experienced as domineering by the observers (Jones 2010, 5–7). The role these factors played in the dress of warriors and soldiers has been well researched for feudal societies (for instance Jones 2010) and European soldiers from the seventeenth century onwards (Abler 1999). The dress of ancient warriors/soldiers has generated less research until now, exceptions include several inquiries into Bronze Age warrior dress (see Treherne 1995; Kristiansen and Larsson 2005, 225, 227–8).

Generally, it can be stated that in most societies where warriors and/or soldiers had a high status, weapons and equipment – and among them especially the sword – were markers of that status (see for instance James 1997, 19; Rubin 2006, 398, James 2011, 18–21; Loveluck 2013, 100-4). In addition, a host of other visual signals could symbolise the status of the warrior/soldier, including permanent body modifications such as tattoos and piercings, or less permanent ones such as hairstyles and body paintings. Dress items and a number of fairly arbitrary objects are also known to have symbolised warrior/soldier status (an example is the five symbols of the Sikh warrior caste, see Dhavan 2011, 6, 142). Only a few of these objects can be identified in the archaeological record, while body posture, language and gestures only turn up obliquely in written sources.

In Roman society, dress and jewellery were among the most commonly used markers of social identity (Rothe 2009, 9). Different items of dress were used to mark social positions, such as different versions of mantles (*toga, pallium, stola*), the decoration of the tunic (*clavi*) or different shoes (*calcei*). Items of jewellery, or rather the material from which they were made (gold, iron), also indicated a person's social status and rank.

The use of items of dress to mark social rank and position has another aspect besides their direct connection with the wearer, namely that they can be removed (Reinhard 2006, 115; Peoples and Bailey 2010, 260). This is useful when the individual wants to assume a different situational identity for a time – e.g. a warrior/soldier may wish to act as a priest. But it is also practical if a social group wants to exclude one of their members, as the public 'di-vestment' of his/her marker dress items is a socially very effective way of symbolising this exclusion. This practice is known for the Roman military belt and was called *discingere* (de-belt). It was used as punishment,

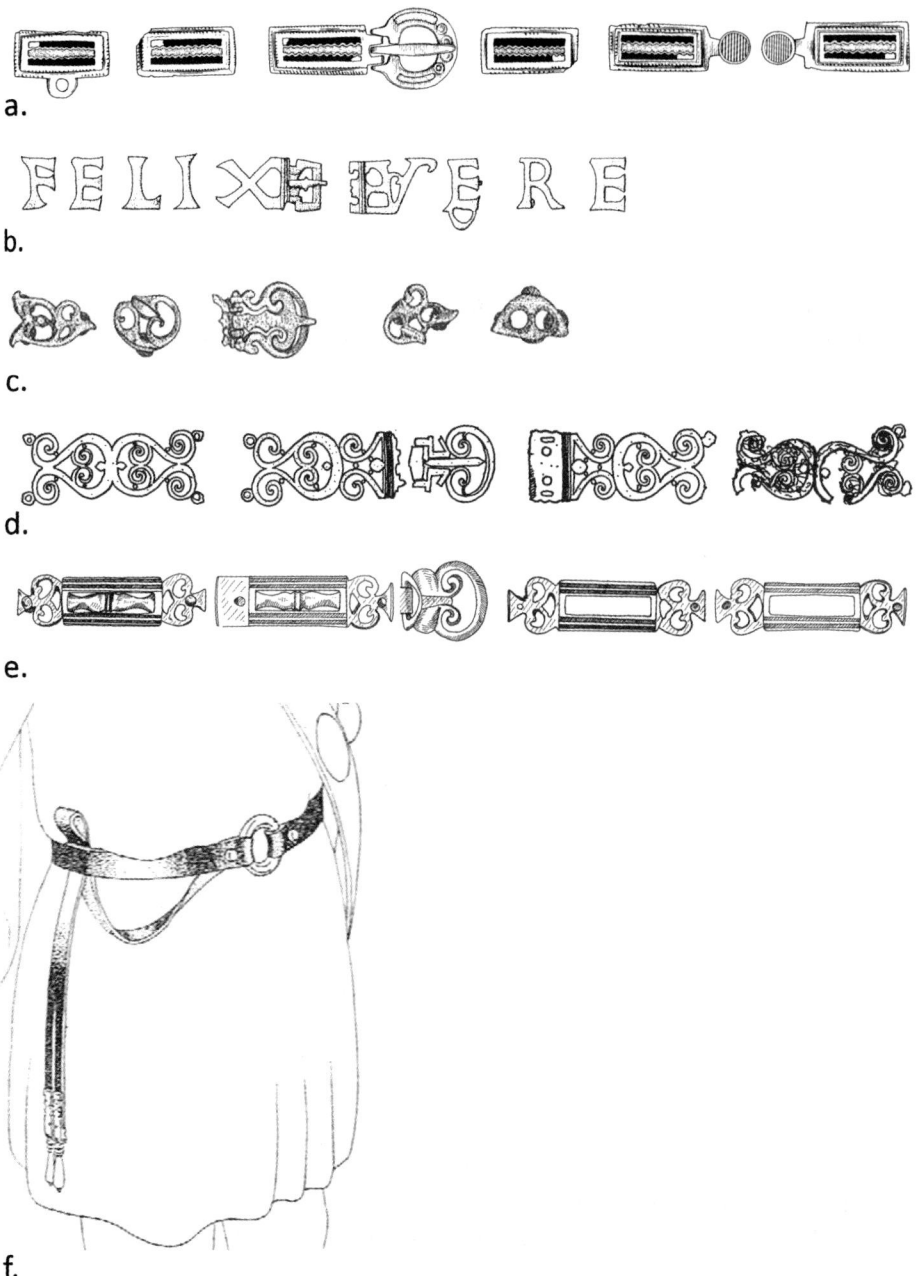

Fig. 5.3: Belt-sets, various dates: a. Chichester, second-third century (after Down/Rule 1971, fig. 5.18); b. Lyon, second-third century (after Bishop and Coulston 2006, fig. 101); c. Faimingen, second-third century (after Müller 1999, pl. 51); d. Neuburg an der Donau, second-third century (after Hübner 1963, fig. 4); e. Lechinta de Mures, second-third century (after Petculescu 1995, pl. 7); f. reconstruction of a third century ring buckle belt (after James 2004, fig. 31a).

with taking away the belt for a certain amount of time – usually a day – used for lesser infractions, while it was taken away permanently at a dishonourable discharge (Livius, XXVII, 13, 9; Frontinus, Stratagemata IV, I, 26–7, 43; Valerius Maximus II, 7, 9; Plutarch Luc. 15; Sueton Octavian 24).

The military belt as a status symbol

The genesis of soldiers as a recognisable social group within Roman society was a side effect of the increasing professionalisation of the Roman army – originally an army of conscript citizens (Alston 2007, 178, 180). While this development had its roots in the second century BC, it gained strength and speed only in the last years of the Roman Republic and was concluded under Augustus, who codified the regulations under which the soldiers served. After his reforms, the army consisted of long-term professional soldiers, commanded by an officer class of senatorial and equestrian rank. The career of the latter was a long line of alternating military and civilian offices in the name of the Emperor (Goldsworthy 2003, 76–81). By the end of the Augustan period, the Roman army had evolved to form a distinct society within the larger society of the Empire (Gilliver 2007, 184–5). This separate society included the professional soldiers – from the raw recruit up to the rank of centurion – signing up for 25 years of service, but not the officer class, who changed between military and civilian assignments.

In Roman law, soldiers were distinguished from civilians by the right to wear arms (especially a sword) at all times and in public, with the exception of the city of Rome itself (Brunt 1976). Civilians were only allowed to wear weapons in vaguely defined exceptional cases, such as while travelling or hunting (Dig. 48.6.1 Marcianus). The separation of the soldiers from the rest of Roman society was cemented by special legal privileges and obligations, but also marked by the guarantee of regular pay, a minimum supply of food, clothing and shelter as well as medical treatment. The distinctness of the social group of the soldiers in contrast to the rest of Roman society was felt and commented upon by civilians, as is proven by several satires (Apuleius, Metamorphosis IX, 39; Juvenal Satires XVI).

In modern sociological terms, a *total institution* describes an institution in which the individual is forced to stay, has hardly any contact with the outside world and all aspects of his life are controlled by that institution (for instance a prison or a psychiatric hospital). A *quasi-total institution*, on the other hand differs from this in that the individuals work and live together, socialising with each other by choice even when off-duty, while still enjoying personal freedom and the possibility to socialise with individuals from outside the institution (Ashford and Meal 1989, 28). In that sense, the Roman army was a '*quasi-total institution*', in which the soldiers spent most days having close and daily contact with their co-soldiers, whom they also often saw socially in their free time. During the long and harsh initial training, recruits were quickly and completely integrated into the community of the '*commilitones*', internalising the formal rules and regulations of the service as well as the more informal social norms and rules. Haynes has emphasised the importance of routine in the process he terms 'incorporation' into the Roman army, using the social concept of *habitus* to explain the cultural transformation a recruit underwent (Haynes 2013, 167).

The social identity of the men who served as Roman soldiers was strongly shaped by their status as soldiers and affiliation to this status was marked by external symbols (Reinhard 2006, 115; Peoples and Bailey 2010, 260). The most important of these external symbols were the weapons and armour of the soldiers, but they were only worn during campaign or exercise. The soldier's everyday costume did not include cumbersome items like spears or armour, helmets and shields. It was reduced to the main weapon of the soldier, the sword, with the frequent supplement of a dagger (Speidel 2009, 241–3).

Both the written sources, and the reliefs and statuary prove however, that soldiers were recognisable as members of their social group even then. All Roman soldiers – be they the citizen soldiers of the legionary units or soldiers without citizen status in the auxiliary units – usually wore a belted tunic, nailed sandals and a long, heavy cloak, fixed on the right shoulder with a brooch (see Figs. 5.1 and 5.3), though this custom should not be mistaken as a uniform (Hoss in press). Among the truly distinguishing factors of the soldier's dress were the mantle/cloak (*sagum*) and the nailed sandals (*caligae*), both of them proverbial for soldiers: while '*saga sumere*' (putting on the *sagum*) was used in the sense of 'going to war', soldiers are regularly described as *caligati* or as serving in *caligae* (Gilliam 1946, 171 (37), 183 (43); Speidel 2009, 243). Of even greater symbolic importance was the military belt, a fact affirmed by both the written sources and the stereotypical depiction of the belt on soldier's gravestones (see Figs. 5.1 and 5.3). The belt obtained this importance by its unity with the sword hanging from it (Hoss 2013, 321). The sword was the main weapon of the Roman soldier and the focal point of his military honour (James 2011, 16–28). Objects of such significance are commonly richly decorated in order to visualise their importance (Swift 2009, 4). Because the sword itself was worn in a sheath, and the sheath was fixed to the belt to carry it, both sheath and belt were seen as belonging to the sword, the three items forming a unit.

Moreover, when a sword is sheathed, only the hilt is visible of the sword itself. While some rare types of Roman sword hilts, for instance the third-century hilts in the form of eagle heads (Miks 2007, 208–11), were quite ornate, most were largely functional and offered little room for decoration. The restrictions on the visible decoration of the sword resulted in both the sheath and the belt being the focus of decoration marking the sword. The symbolic status of the sword was thus projected onto the sheath and the belt, making the latter an important identifying dress item for soldiers.

This use of the belt as a status marker was reflected in the abundant metal decoration that became common from the late first century BC onwards (see Fig. 5.1 and Fig. 5.2a–b): elaborate buckles, metal mounts, strap-ends and other attachments were fixed to the belt, which made the belt both eye-catching and heavy. If we take the belts and apron worn by Publius Flavoleuis Cordus (Fig. 5.1) as an example, the total weight, excluding the sword and dagger, easily exceeded a kilo (Hoss in prep.). This was a lot of additional weight for a soldier, who also had to carry about 45kg of weapons, equipment and food during a march (see Roth 1999, 71–7). As the belt and apron decoration had no technical function, the compensation for this disadvantage must have been a very important social function.

The only exception in the use of the belt as a marker of the status of a soldier were the Roman cavalrymen, who wore belts with belt buckles, but without metal mounts or 'aprons' during the first and most of the second century. They seem to have adopted belts decorated with mounts only by the late second century, after which they appear in the same belts as the other soldiers (see Hoss 2010).

As we have seen, by the mid-second century AD, the sword was no longer worn on a belt around the waist, but instead on a shoulder-belt. Interestingly, the symbolic importance of the belt as a dress item for the Roman soldier was not transferred to the shoulder-belt, where the sword – the focal point the military honour – was now worn. It is an indication of the sense of tradition in the Roman army and of the value the military belt had attained as a symbol by then, that the military belt worn around the waist remained the key marker of military status and even increased in importance in succeeding centuries. This increase is demonstrated by the adoption of the belt by the military elite during the third century AD: reliefs on a number of large third-century marble sarcophagi originally from Rome depict scenes from the hunt or the battle. These show high officers from the Roman aristocracy with the typical military belt with a ring-shaped buckle (Andreae 1980, Cat. No. 28, 65, 122, 128 192; Künzl 2010, Figs. 72, 75). Similar belts are depicted as worn by the emperors on several Sassanid triumphal reliefs (Hoss 2015).

The significance of the traditional belt as a symbol of 'being a soldier' continued well into Late Antiquity as is demonstrated by the symbolic act of Christian soldier-saints openly refusing to remain in the army by the symbolic gesture of throwing off their military belt in public (Woods 1993, 55–60). The symbolic value of the waist-belt as a marker of the warrior/soldier even extended beyond the borders of the Roman Empire into *barbaricum*, where numerous elite male graves contain belts decorated with metal mounts and belt buckles (see Abegg-Wigg and Lau 2014). The symbolism of the belt proved to be enduring under the successors of the Roman Empire both in the West and East and waist-belts decorated with metal mounts remained an important signal of martial masculinity well into the Early Middle Ages (Fehr 1999, Schulze-Dörrlamm 2002, Marzinzik 2003, Brather 2008).

In its importance as a transmitter of a univocal message about the wearer's identity and conscious affiliation in Roman society, the military belt is comparable to the Roman *toga* (Wallace-Hadrill 2008, 41–2). While the *toga* characterised a man as a Roman citizen, from the Augustan period onwards, the military belt characterised its wearer – from the simple *miles* to the *centurio* – as a soldier. It was the privilege of those who were or had been in military service, both as soldiers exposed to actual warfare (*militia armata*) and as civil servants detailed to various administrative tasks in the Empire (*militia officialis*). As Speidel has clearly shown, the latter also were serving as soldiers in the *militia* with all the rights of soldiers granted to them, including wearing the military belt (Speidel 2006). The belt was important in the formation, definition and experience of the social community of the soldiers and expressed their group identity in a socially appropriate way.

The demonstration of this group identity worked in two ways: civilians seeing a soldier with such a belt directly identified its wearer as a soldier, but the soldiers themselves were also re-committed to their group by seeing a belt similar to theirs on other soldiers (Sommer 2012, 258–9). For this identification to work, the different belts did not need to look completely identical, it was sufficient if the different elements were reasonably similar to be recognised as part of the same idiom.

Additional messages of the military belt

While the main statement of the military belt – that its wearer was a soldier or a veteran – was inherent to it, its decoration with metal mounts could also convey additional messages. Among them is the relative wealth of the soldiers – a leather belt with metal mounts was always more expensive than the textile belt that held the civilian's tunic. In addition to that, the rank of the soldier seems to have been signalled by the value of the metal chosen for the mounts, with silver reserved for the centurions.

The choice of motifs for the decoration of the mounts also expressed additional messages, but most were highly stylised and are difficult to recognise. During the first century AD, the decorations included stylised depictions of Jupiter's bolt of lighting (Fig. 5.2b, on the left and in the middle of the middle plate), symbolising the support of the highest god of state, or stylised laurels as symbols of victory. Equally stylised are the shield bosses that were preferred in Flavian times (Figs. 5.2d–e). Directly recognisable are the Lupa Romana giving suck to Romulus and Remus, a depiction used as a sort of coat of arms of Rome, and the emperor's head surrounded by *cornucopiae*, suggestive of the riches to be expected by his reign (Fig. 5.2c). These motifs resemble similar ones on sword sheaths, which formed an iconographic unit with the belt, but have no direct connection to the depictions on helmets and armour, which mainly show figures of gods (Hoss in prep.; Schamper 2015.). They are, however, similar in that both the depictions of gods on the arms and armour and the symbols used on the belt plates are often connected to (a) state deities (Jupiter, Victory), (b) symbols of the state (Lupa Romana, emperor) or (c) war (victory laurels, shield bosses).

More difficult to understand are the decorations preferred during the second and third centuries, many of which are stylised forms of tendrils (see Figs. 5.3c–d). Other forms demonstrate a different sort of religiosity from the first-century promotion of state gods, namely magical protection. They combine apotropaic signs (in this case, the pelta, Fig. 5.3e) with written wishes of wellbeing, like *Utere felix* ('wear in happiness'), a wish fairly common on various small personal items at the time (see Fig. 5.3b, see Hoss 2006). These motifs are comparable to those on the mounts of the shoulder-belts, which by now formed an iconographic unit with the belt. They are, however, different from the motifs on helmets and armour, which combine apotropaic signs (snakes) with figures of gods, albeit from a wider pantheon than in the first century (see Schamper 2015). The conspicuous absence of state gods and the preference for other forms of religiosity are the only connections between the belt sets on one hand and the armour and helmet on the other.

On a meta-level, the decorated belt mirrored two elements of the Roman soldier's equipment and enhanced them. One is the visual effect of shining metal surfaces, which were quite common in soldier's equipment, as the armour, helmet and greaves were made mainly from metal. In contrast to this, male civilian dress was almost without metal elements, with the exception of a brooch. The other was the characteristic sound emitted by the equipment. As almost all parts of the Roman soldier's equipment were made from a combination of leather and metal parts, the slightest movement of the wearer produced two kinds of sound: the creaking of leather and the clanging of metal. This soundscape was characteristic for soldiers on the move and differentiated them from civilians who, as their dress consisted of a tunic and mantle with many folds, must have been characterised by the sound of a textile rustle. Both the visual characteristics (shiny metal) and the soundscape (creaking and jingling) were picked up and enhanced by the military belt. The combined creaking and jangling of the equipment and the apron, plus the noise of the hobnailed sandals on paved streets must have made a very impressive soundscape when a whole unit of soldiers marched by (Bishop and Coulston 2006, 110). But the apron made even a single soldier audibly recognisable, even when he was not wearing his full equipment, but just his everyday apparel.

Even after the apron had been given up, the soundscape of creaking and jangling was still typical for Roman soldiers. From the mid-second century AD onwards, the belt strap between the holes for the buckle pin and the end was very long and split into two straps, from which two free-swinging hangers fell (see Fig. 5.3f). The straps usually were tucked under the belt on the right side and hung from there to the knee, also jangling with every step (James 2006, 61). The sound of these straps was probably less impressive than that of the apron, but the continuity of audible signals of the presence of soldiers is worth remarking upon.

Fashion

As we have seen, the belt mounts changed considerably in appearance over the three centuries under investigation (see Figs. 5.2–3). These changes were universal: the belt mounts of any given period demonstrate a surprising similarity throughout the whole

Roman Empire, from Hadrian's Wall to Egypt and from Pannonia to Morocco. But this similarity is by no means uniformity. Although the basic design of contemporary belt mounts and buckles is frequently very similar, the execution is almost always slightly different, according to the means and abilities of the maker and the financial resources of the buyer. While some pieces undoubtedly come from the same maker and sometimes even the very same casting-mould, most were produced in the far-flung corners of the Empire with the available local experience and to the craftsmen's own standards.

A question raised by the similarity of these designs of the decorations is their instigation: who chose the designs – the individual soldiers or a central authority, for instance the commander of a unit or even central administration in Rome itself? It seems likely that most of the decoration was the choice of the soldiers themselves, as the belts were their personal possessions. Papyri and literary sources prove that, in joining the army, one set of standard equipment was given to the soldiers out of a unit stock depot (*armamentarium*, Breeze et al. 1976, 93). The soldiers paid for this equipment through deductions from their salary, which probably helped to ensure they took good care of it (Tacitus, Annales, 1,17). A similar system seems viable for the military belts. As with the other equipment, it was possible to add to this stock and buy your own, perhaps reselling your old equipment to the unit (Breeze et al. 1976, 94). Tacitus writes about some soldiers who gave their belts in lieu of money, which proves that they must have been both valuable and the personal property of the soldiers in question (Tacitus, Histora, I, 57). The finds of buckles and mounts of military belts in graves further prove this point, as the presence of belts in graves suggest that the objects were the personal possession of the deceased (Mackensen 1987, 158–9). This makes it very likely that the choice of decoration – as with other items of military equipment – lay in the owner's hands.

Another reason to assume that the soldiers themselves largely instigated the design changes is the fact that the Roman army did not have the possibility – in terms of organisation and production – to manufacture such vast amounts of similar items (Hoss in press). Uniformity in dress and equipment was also seen as contrary to morale, as the competition of Roman soldiers amongst each other on the battlefield was based on their recognisability (Hoss in press). The Roman army simply had neither the means nor the inclination to make their soldiers look similar in every way.

The changes between the different overall designs appear sudden in the archaeological record, but they were most likely more gradual in reality. One important fact driving the seemingly abrupt appearance of certain belt fashions was war itself and the loss of soldiers and equipment connected to it. After a long campaign involving heavy losses, new recruits had to be found and equipped. These new recruits or new units were mostly furnished with new equipment, the old armour and weapons usually having been stripped off their dead colleagues by the enemy on the field. When found, this new material then often seems simultaneous, even if it found its way into the archaeological record over a period of several decades. This is because our dating methods, despite recent advancements, are still rather rough. When determining the date of belt mounts, we are very lucky if we can be more precise than a quarter century.

We have thus to conclude that the changes in belt decoration were motivated by the soldiers themselves and that they were motivated not by technical needs, but correspond with what can be described as fashion changes.

Earlier research on fashion presumed that the phenomenon started to appear during the fourteenth and fifteenth centuries, assuming that while older societies used dress as a mode of communication, they did not know fashion (Davis 1992, 28; Belfanti 2009; Reinhard 2006, 120). As fashion seemed to be characterised by fast changes that are not motivated by necessity, the comparatively slow changes in dress observed in ancient societies did not fit the pattern. But this confuses the phenomenon of fashion with its mode of transport, namely the possibility of visual contact with the new fashion. The pace of fashion is dictated by the pace of the dissemination of pictures or people displaying these fashions. Because of the slower dissemination of these in ancient societies, fashion changes may have been slower. But they can be discerned nonetheless, for instance in the changes of the Empresses' coiffures that were disseminated through their portraits on coins and copied by elegant ladies throughout the Empire (Mannsperger 1998, 29–75). Other studies could demonstrate the workings of fashion in Late Antique and Early Medieval societies (Brather 2008, 249).

Fashion changes in Roman military belt decorations were most likely occasioned by the fact that while soldiers rarely changed units, their centurions were transferred to other units quite often, taking the newest styles with them. In addition, long campaigns, in which larger armies composed of several legions and other units would meet, also had a large influence on the belt fashions of their time. Here, the soldiers from different units would spend months or years camping, marching and fighting together. Accordingly, theatres of war were hotbeds for the development and spreading of new belt fashions.

The competitive Roman honour culture, identified by Speidel (1994, 386–7) and Lendon (1997, 249–51) as a main driving force behind the fighting power of both individual Roman soldiers and whole units, ensured that each unit and each individual soldier would constantly strive to outdo the others in achievements, a fact that was utilised by the command in having units work competitively against each other (Lendon 2005, 255). Honour could be won by the competent execution of difficult tasks like the building of a bridge, but the main sources for honour were, of course, feats of daring on the battlefield. Next to official decorations such as *torques*, *armillae* or *phalerae*, which were only worn during parades (Maxfield 1981), the visual outward expression of the soldier's honour was the possession of splendid arms and armour, decorated and polished to a high finish. Together with the sword, the sword-belt can be described as an expression of such an honour culture.

Body posture

As we have seen above, dress is used to promote characteristic body postures. Dominant male dress tends to promote and emphasise a straight and erect posture, with the shoulders back, the breast thrust forward and the waist pronounced. This posture enlarges and widens the upper body visually and this effect is used to demonstrate dominant power not only by men, but also various male animals (Davies 2005, 122). A Roman example of the workings of dress on posture is the *toga* (Davies 2005). A *toga* consisted of a single piece of wool cloth about 6m long and 2.5m wide. This very heavy piece of cloth was draped about a man in various fashionable manners, but not fastened. It needed two helpers to dress in a *toga*, because the correct fall of the folds was highly important. As the folds tended to slide during rapid movement, the *toga* ensured that its wearer assumed an erect posture and measured movements (Goette 2013, 42–7).

As we have also seen earlier, the Roman military belt was quite heavy and experiments with wearing reconstructed Roman military belts have shown that the weight of the belt tends to influence the wearer's posture. It made running very difficult and promoted a posture with feet planted wide during standing, and a very characteristic wide-legged, swaying walk (Bishop and Coulston 2006, 254; James 2006, 257). This manner of standing and walking is also known from individuals wearing various modern belts, some of which carry heavy equipment (carpenter-belts) or weapons (pistol-belts) or a combination of both (police-belts).

The body posture of Roman soldiers on their gravestones is very similar, with most displaying the typical stance with feet spread the width of the hips. Ancient literature also confirms that Roman soldiers had a specific body posture characterised by a swaggering walk, and completed by an arrogant pose and brash insolence, often used to intimidate civilians (see Apuleius, Metamorphoses IX, 39). As the authors of these descriptions were upper-class males espousing a set of urban/civic values, it is possible that their critique was a social commentary on lower-class males using a martial stance to demonstrate their power over civilians (Hoss in press).

The perceived arrogance of the posture is heightened by a gesture that emerges on gravestones from the third century AD, in which the soldier holds the long strap ends of the belt in his right hand (Fig. 5.4). According to Coulston it is likely that this is a depiction of a gesture that was visible daily on the streets of Roman garrison towns, in which the soldiers swung the long strap ends of their belts around. These ends were split and each decorated with a long and heavy copper-alloy hanger, which clicked against each other. The arrogant menace exuded by this gesture is evident and emphasises the importance the soldiers had achieved as a social group by then (Coulston 2005, 151).

Conclusion

We can thus summarise that the Roman military belt was inextricably linked to the genesis of the professional soldier in the Roman army during the early Augustan

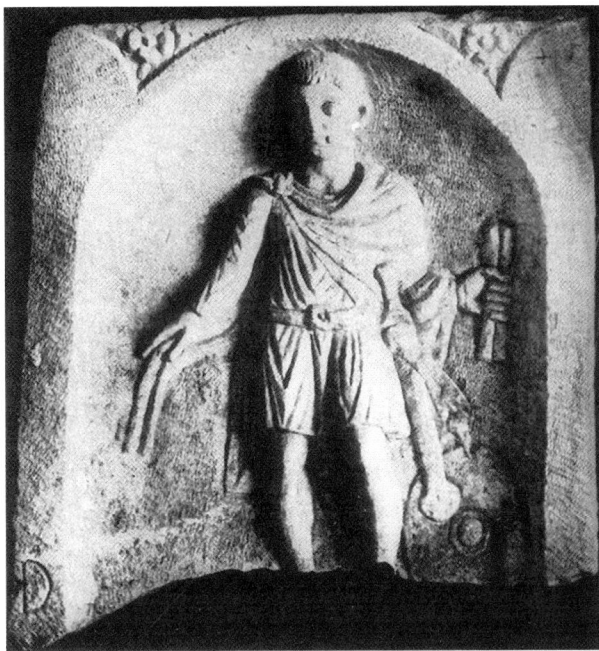

Fig. 5.4: Funerary monument of an unknown soldier in Istanbul (third century AD), displaying the end of his belt (after Pfuhl/Möbius 1978, cat. no. 315, pl. 56).

age in the last decades of the first century BC. From this time until the end of Late Antiquity it served as a status symbol, signifying that its wearer was a Roman soldier or a veteran. In this function it was an important tool in defining and experiencing the social community of the soldiers, evoking positive feelings of belonging to this particular social group, construing itself as superior to others.

The emergence of the status symbol of the 'military belt' thus not only took place a good 300 years earlier than is often thought, but the reason for this development is now clearly to be sought in the creation of a new and privileged social group, which soon acquired status markers. This connection also better explains the importance of the military belt in Late Antiquity.

In addition to its main message of social status, the material of the belt decoration could transmit information about the rank of the soldier, while the meaning of the highly stylised designs are more difficult to decipher. Those that are recognisable either refer to war or demonstrate attachment to divine protection, an understandable desire on the battlefield. A visible change occurs in the choice of gods asked for protection between the first and the second to third centuries AD, with state gods such as Jupiter preferred in the first century, while the latter two centuries are marked by preference for a more magical approach to protection. This very likely marks a change in the Roman army's successes: while the army had been (mostly) victorious during the first century, it was markedly less so during the second and third centuries AD. This was occasioned by various causes, whose discussion is beyond the scope of this paper. However, it seems likely, that the general instability and especially the heightened personal danger of dying on the battlefield prompted the soldiers to try their luck with all supernatural forces and not restrict themselves to the gods representing the Roman state.

Because of the impossibility to produce such vast amounts of similar belt mounts by order and the fact that the soldiers owned their belts, it has to be assumed that the simultaneous changes in belt design, occurring about once every quarter century, were initiated by the soldiers themselves. They have been shown to be an expression of fashion, which moved slower in ancient societies due to the slower dissemination of pictures and people which made viewing (and thus following) a new fashion possible. The weight of the belt on the soldier also had an effect on his body postures, promoting an erect and wide-legged stance that was socially interpreted as domineering.

The Roman military belt was thus both a status symbol, transmitting a univocal message about the wearer's identity and conscious affiliation, as well as a dress item that carried additional messages of rank and belief. Its decoration was influenced by fashion and its weight manipulated the body posture of its wearer.

Bibliography

Abegg-Wigg, A. and Lau, N. (2014) *Kammergräber im Barbaricum. Zu Einflüssen und Übergangsphänomenen von der vorrömischen Eisenzeit bis in die Völkerwanderungszeit. Internationale Tagung Schleswig 25.-27. November 2010.* Hamburg, Wachholtz Verlag (Schriften des Archäologischen Landesmuseums Ergänzungsreihe Band 9).

Abler, T. S. (1999) *Hinterland Warriors and Military Dress: European Empires and Exotic Uniforms.* Oxford, Berg.

Alston, R. (2007) The military and politics. In Ph. Sabin, H. van Wees and M. Whitby (eds.) *The Cambridge History of Greek and Roman Warfare, Vol. II*, 176–97. Cambridge, Cambridge University Press.

Anderson, L. M. (2009) The Roman Military Community as Expressed in its Burial Customs during the First to Third Centuries CE. Unpublished Thesis, Brown University.

Andreae, B. (1980) Die römischen Jagdsarkophage. *Die antiken Sarkophagreliefs* 1, 2. Berlin, Mann.

Ashforth, B. E. and Mael, F. (1989) Social identity theory and the organization. *The Academy of Management Review* 14(1), 20–39.

Belfanti, C. M. (2009) The civilization of fashion: at the origins of a Western social institution. *Journal of Social History* 43(2), 261–83.

Bishop, M. C. and Coulston J. C. N. (2006) *Roman Military Equipment from the Punic wars to the fall of Rome.* Oxford, Oxbow Books.

Böhme, H. W. (1974) *Germanische Grabfunde des 4. bis 5. Jh. n. Chr. zwischen unterer Elbe und Loire.* Munich, C. H. Beck'sche Verlagsbuchhandlung (Münchner Beiträge zur Vor- und Frühgeschichte 19).

Brather, S. (2008) Kleidung, Bestattung, Identität – Die Präsentation sozialer Rollen im frühen Mittelalter. In S. Brather (ed.) *Zwischen Spätantike und Frühmittelalter. Archäologie des 4. bis 7. Jh. n. Chr. im Westen*, 237–73. Berlin, Walter de Gruyter (Reallexikon Germanischer Altertumskunde Ergänzungsband 57).

Breeze, D. J., Close-Brooks, J. and Graham Ritchie, J. N. (1976) Soldiers' Burials at Camelon, Stirlingshire, 1922 and 1957. *Britannia* 7, 73–95.

Brunt, P. A. (1976), Did Rome disarm her citizens? *Phoenix* 29, 260–70.

Bullinger, H. (1969) *Spätantike Gürtelbeschläge: Typen, Herstellung, Trageweise und Datierung*. Brügge, De Tempel.

Collins, R. (2008) Identity in the frontier: theory and multiple community interfacing. In C. M. Fenwick, M. Wiggins and D. Wythe (eds.) *TRAC 2007: Proceedings of the Seventh Annual Theoretical Roman Archaeology Conference, London 2007*, 45–52. Oxford, Oxbow Books.

Coulston, J. C. N. (2005) Military identity and personal self-identity in the Roman army. In L. de Ligt, E. A. Hemelrijk and H. W. Singor (eds.) *Roman Rule and Civic Life: Local and Regional Perspectives. Impact of Empire 4*, 133–52. Amsterdam, J. C. Gieben.

Davis, F. (1992) *Fashion, Culture and Identity*. Chicago, University of Chicago Press.

Davies, G. (2005) What made the Roman Toga *virilis*? In L. Cleland, M. Harlow and L. Llewellyn-Jones (eds.) *The Clothed Body in the Ancient World*, 121–30. Oxford, Oxbow Books.

Dharvan, P. (2011) *When Sparrows Became Hawks: The Making of the Sikh Warrior Tradition, 1699-1799*. Oxford, Oxford University Press.

Down, A. and Rule, M. (1971) *Chichester Excavations I*. Oxford, Philimore & Co Ltd.

Fehr, H. (1999) Zur Deutung der Prunkgürtelsitte der jüngeren Merowingerzeit. Das Verhältnis von Waffenbeigabe und Gürtelbeigabeanhand der Männergräber von Schretzheim und Kirchheim/Ries. In S. Brather, Chr. Bücker and M. Hoeper (eds.), *Archäologie als Sozialgeschichte. Studien zu Siedlung, Wirtschaft und Gesellschaft im frühgeschichtlichen Mitteleuropa. Festschrift Heiko Steuer*, 105–111. Rahden/Westfalen, M. Leidorf (Studia Honoria 9).

Fischer, T. (2011) *Die Armee der Caesaren: Archäologie und Geschichte*. Regensburg, Verlag Friedrich Pustet.

Gilliam, J. F. (1946) Milites Caligati. *Transactions and Proceedings of the American Philological Association* 77, 183–91. Reprinted in: Gilliam, J. F. 1986, *Roman Army Papers*, 43–191. Amsterdam, J. C. Gieben (MAVORS II).

Gilliver, K. (2007) The Augustean reform and the structure of the imperial army. In P. Erdkamp (ed.) *A Companion to the Roman Army*, 183–200. Oxford, Blackwell.

Goette, H. R. (2013) Die römische 'Staatstracht' – toga, tunica und calcei. In M. Tellenbach, R. Schulz und A. Wieczorek (eds.) *Die Macht der Toga. Dress Code im Römischen Weltreich. Begleitband zur Sonderausstellung im Römer-Pelizaeus-Museum Hildesheim 20. April-8. September 2013*, 39–52. Regensburg, Roemer- und Pelizaeus-Museum (Publikation der Reiss-Engelhorn-Mussen 56).

Goldsworthy, A. (2003) *The Complete Roman Army*. London, Thames and Hudson.

Haynes, I. (2013) *Blood of the Provinces. The Roman Auxilia and the Making of Provincial Society from Augustus to the Severans*. Oxford, Oxford University Press.

Hogg, M. A., Terry, D. J. and White, K. M. (1995) A tale of two theories: a critical comparison of identity theory with social identity theory. *Social Psychology Quarterly* 58(4), 255–69.

Hoss, S. (2006) VTERE FELIX und MNHNΩN – Zu den Gürteln mit Buchstabenbeschlägen. *Archäologisches Korrezpondenzblatt* 2006/2, 237–53.

Hoss, S. (2010) The military belts of the equites. In H.-J. Schalles and A. W. Busch (eds.) *Waffen in Aktion. Akten der XVI. International Roman Military Equipment Conference*, 313–22. Mainz am Rhein, Philipp von Zabern (Xantener Berichte 16).

Hoss, S. (2011) The Roman military belt. In M.-L. Nosch and H. Koefoed (ed.) *Wearing the Cloak. Dressing the Soldier in Roman Times*, 29–44. Oxford, Oxbow Books (Ancient Textiles Series 10).

Hoss, S. (2013) A theoretical approach to Roman military belts. In M. Sanader, A. Rendić-Miočević, D. Tončinić and I. Radman-Livaja (eds.) *Proceedings of the XVII Roman Military Equipment Conference Zagreb 24-27th May 2010*, 317–26. Zagreb, Filozofski fakultet, Odsjek za arheologiju.

Hoss, S. (2015). The origin of the ring buckle belt and the Persian wars of the 3rd century. In L. Vagalinski and N. Sharankov (eds.) *Limes XXII. Proceedings of the 22nd International Congress of Roman Frontier Studies Ruse, Bulgaria, September 2012* (Bulletin of the National Archaeological Institute XLII), 319–26. Sofia, NIAM-BAS.

Hoss, S. (2016) Dressing the Roman soldier. In X. Pauli Jensen and Th. Grane (eds.), *Imitation and Inspiration. Proceedings of the 18th International Roman Military Equipment Conference held in Copenhagen, Denmark, 9th-14th June 2013*, Journal of Roman Military Equipment Studies 17, 115–120.

Hoss, S. (in press), *CINGULUM MILITARE. Studien zum römischen Soldatengürtel des 1. bis 3. Jh. n. Chr.* Rahden/Westfalen, Verlag Marie Leidorf.

Hübener, W. (1963/64) Zu den provinzialrömischen Waffenfunden. Saalburg-Jahrbuch XXI, 20–25.

James, E. (1997) The militarisation of Roman society, 400–700. In A. N. Jørgensen and B. L. Clausen (eds.) *Military Aspects of Scandinavian Society in a European Perspective, AD 1-1300*, 19–24. Copenhagen, Danish National Museum (Publications from the National Museum studies in Archaeology and History 2).

James, S. (2004) *The Excavations at Dura-Europos conducted by Yale University and the French Academy of Inscriptions and Letters 1928 to 1937. Final report VII: The Arms and Amour and other Military Equipment.* London, British Museum Press.

James, S. (2006) Engendering change in our understanding of the structure of Roman military communities. *Archaeological Dialogues* 13(1), 31–6.

James, S. (2011) *Rome and the Sword: How Warriors and Weapons Shaped Roman History.* London, Thames and Hudson.

Jones, R. W. (2010) *Bloodied Banners: Martial Display on the Medieval Battlefield.* Woodbridge, Boydell Press.

Kristiansen, K. and Larsson, Th. B., eds. (2005) *The Rise of Bronze Age Society: Travels, Transmissions and Transformations.* Cambridge, Cambridge University Press.

Künzl, E. (2010) *Der Traum vom Imperium. Der Ludovisisarkophag - Grabmal eines Feldherren Roms.* Mainz, Schnell and Steiner.

Lendon, J. E. (1997) *Empire of Honour. The Art of Government in the Roman World.* Oxford, Clarendon Press.

Lendon, J. E. (2005) *Soldiers and Ghosts. A History of Battle in Classical Antiquity.* New Haven, Yale University Press.

Loveluck, C. (2013) *Northwest Europe in the Early Middle Ages, c. AD 600-1150: A Comparative Archaeology.* Cambridge, Cambridge University Press.

Mackensen, M. (1987) *Die frühkaiserzeitliche Kleinkastelle bei Nersingen und Burlafingen an der oberen Donau.* Munich, Beck (Münchener Beiträge zur Vor- und Frühgeschichte 41).

Mannsperger, M. (1998) *Frisurenkunst und Kunstfrisur. Die Haarmode der römischen Kaiserinnen von Livia bis Sabina.* Bonn, Habelt.

Marzinzik, S. (2003) *Early Anglo-Saxon Belt Buckles (Late 5th to Early 8th Centuries A.D.) Their classification and context.* Oxford, Archaeopress (British Archaeological Reports, British Series 357).

Maxfield, V. A. (1981) *The Military Decorations of the Roman Army.* London, Batsfield.

Miks, Chr. (2007) *Studien zur römischen Schwertbewaffnung in der Kaiserzeit.* Rahden, Marie Leidorf (Kölner Studien zur Archäologie der römischen Provinzen 8).

Morel, J.-M. A. W. and Bosman, A. V. A. J. (1989) An early Roman burial in Velsen I. In C. van Driel-Murray (ed.), *Roman Military Equipment: the sources of evidence. Proceedings of the fifth Roman military equipment conference,* BAR International series 476. Oxford, Archeopress.

Müller, M. (1999) Die römischen Grabfunde von Phoebiana – Faimingen. Limesforschungen 26, Mainz, von Zabern.

Petculescu, L. (1995) Military Equipment Graves in Roman Dacia. *Journal of Roman Military Equipment Studies* 6, 105–145.

Peoples, J. G. and Bailey, G. A. (2010) *Humanity: An Introduction to Cultural Anthropology.* Belmont, Wadsworth.

Pfuhl, E. and Möbius, H. (1978) *Die ostgriechischen Grabreliefs.* Mainz, Von Zabern.

Reinhard, W. (2006) *Lebensformen Europas. Eine historische Kulturanthropologie.* Munich, C. H. Beck.

Roth, J. P. (1999) *The Logistics of the Roman Army at War (264 B.C.-A.D. 235).* Leiden, Brill.

Rothe, U. (2009) *Dress and Cultural Identity in the Rhine-Moselle Region of the Roman Empire.* Oxford: Archaeopress (British Archaeological Reports, International Series 2038).

Rubin, M. (2006) 'Identities'. In R. Horrox and M. Ormrod (eds.) *A Social History of England, 1200–1500*, 483–512. Cambridge, Cambridge University Press.
Schamper, J. (2015) *Studien zu Paraderüstungsteilen und anderen verzierten Waffen der Römischen Kaiserzeit*. Rahden/Westfalen, Marie Leidorf (Kölner Studien zur Archäologie der römischen Provinzen 12).
Schulze-Dörrlamm, M. (2002) *Byzantinische Gürtelschnallen und Gürtelbeschläge im Römisch-Germanischen Zentralmuseum. Teil I: Die Schnallen ohne Beschläg, mit Laschenbeschläg und mit festem Beschläg des 5. bis 7. Jahrhunderts*. Mainz, Verlag des Römisch-Germanischen Zentralmuseums (Kataloge vor- und frühgeschichtlicher Altertümer 30, 1).
Sommer, M. (1984) *Die Gürtel und Gürtelbeschläge des 4. und 5. Jahrhunderts im römischen* Reich. Bonn, Institut für Vor- und Frühgeschichte der Rheinischen Friedrich-Wilhelms-Universität (Bonner Hefte zur Vorgeschichte 22).
Sommer, C. M. (2012) Dress and identity – a social psychologist's perspective. In S. Schrenk, K. Vössing and M. Tellenbach (eds.) *Kleidung und Identität in religiösen Kontexten der römischen Kaiserzeit. Altertumswissenschaftliches Kolloquium in Verbindung mit der Arbeitsgruppe 'Kleidung und Religion', Projekt DressID, Rheinische Friedrich-Willhelms-Universität Bonn 30. und 31. Oktober 2009*, 257–63. Regensburg, Schnell and Steiner (Mannheimer Geschichtsblätter Sonderveröffentlichung 4).
Speidel, M. A. (2006) Militia. Zu Sprachgebrauch und Militarisierung in der kaiserzeitlichen Verwaltung. In A. Kolb (ed.) *Herrschaftsstrukturen und Herrschaftspraxis*, 263–8. Berlin, Akademie.
Speidel, M. A. (2009) Dressed for the occasion. Clothes and context in the Roman army. In M. A. Speidel (ed.) *Heer und Herrschaft im römischen Reich der Kaiserzeit*, 235–48. Stuttgart, Franz Steiner Verlag. Also in M.-L. Nosch, ed., (2011) *Wearing the Cloak. Dressing the Soldier in Roman Times*, 1–12. Oxford, Oxbow Books (Ancient Textiles Series 10).
Speidel, M. P. (1994) *Die Denkmäler der Kaiserreiter. Equites Singulares Augusti*. Cologne, Rheinland-Verlag in Kommission bei R. Habelt.
Swift, E. (2000) *Regionality in Dress Accessories in the Late Roman West*. Montagnac, Editions Monique Mergoil (Monographies Instrumentum 11).
Swift, E. (2009) *Style and Function in Roman Decoration. Living with Objects and Interiors*. Farnham, Ashgate.
Treherne, P. (1995) The warrior's beauty: the masculine body and self identity in Bronze-Age Europe. *European Archaeology* 3(1), 105–44.
Ulbert, G. (1969) Das frührömische Kastell Rheingönnheim; die Funde aus den Jahren 1912 und 1913. *Limesforschungen* 9, Berlin, Mann.
Wallace Hadrill, A. (2008) *Rome's Cultural Revolution*. Cambridge, Cambridge University Press.
Woods, D. (1993) The ownership and disposal of military equipment in the Late Roman army. *Journal of Roman Military Equipment Studies* 4, 55–65.

Chapter 6

Middle Anglo-Saxon dress accessories in life and death: expressions of a worldview

Alexandra Knox

Introduction

Dress accessories are universally understood to represent much more than simple decoration or the holding together of garments. Recent work on brooches in the Anglo-Saxon period by the editors of this volume strongly underscores the significance of symbolism, identity and that the wearing of items contributed to the worldview of those participating in certain fashions and stylistic repertoires (Martin 2015; Weetch 2014). Sometimes the meaning of dress accessories can be quite overt: a simple cross design on a brooch dated to the late Anglo-Saxon period (eighth to eleventh centuries AD), when Christianity had become established in Anglo-Saxon England, clearly references the belief system or religious identity of the wearer (Weetch 2014). However, the expression of belief and identity through a dress item by an individual is often less clear cut (e.g. Keefer *et al.* 2010; Petts 2011, 45). For instance, the use of particular animal iconography clearly references a 'worldview' if not an exact belief system but this can be hard to access (e.g. bracteates, see Behr 2000, 25–52). Plenty of brooches, beads and pins, do not, however, appear to directly or immediately reference a particular worldview, or if they do, we have difficulty accessing direct meaning, even in the case of the highly characteristic animal art of the earlier Anglo-Saxon period known as Salin's Style I and II. The particular importance of the dress accessory, with its direct relationship with the body (Martin 2014, 27) and its potential as a participant in defining dividual personhood (Fowler 2004, 7), indicates that in looking to interpret the worldviews of past cultures, dress accessories are a way to access this indistinct sphere. Although the cemetery is the most productive in terms of dress items, and graves can provide additional and detailed contextual information, many dress items are not found in funereal contexts but either come from settlements or have no context at all. How then can we move forward and contextualise and theorise the significance of single dress items or apparent casual losses?

Every object, whether a dress accessory or not, can be seen as having a form of material agency. Chris Tilley has built on the work of art historian Alfred Gell (1998), explaining the importance of artefact agency in the creation of worldviews and social relationships: '(t)hrough making, using, exchanging, consuming, interacting and living with things people make themselves in the process' (Tilley 2006, 61). Dress accessories are the active result of a cultural identity or a belief system. Rather than a reflexive process, however, this bond between person(s) and object(s) is a complicated one. Ian Hodder (2011, 154–77) suggests an inexorable entanglement of relationships, where it is impossible to separate human from thing. The dress accessory, therefore, is a special category as by its very nature it is inseparable from the human individual because it is (nearly always) initially created with the intention of being worn on the body, and contributing to the 'symbolic language' of the body (Mauss 1973, 76; Martin 2014, 27). It also actively takes part in the creation of the identity of the wearer, and rather than expressing identity, the wearing of dress accessories constitutes the activity that embodies the wearer (Fisher and Loren 2003, 228; Martin 2014, 28). When items are found away from their intended purpose – in the settlement rather than the burial – this immediately raises questions regarding their active meaning when physically (if not ideologically) separate from person, and the agency they contain separately to the wearer. It is these meanings in particular that this chapter focuses upon.

If 'things' can be agents, both imbued with and imbuing meaning, then these meanings, effects and relationships can be recorded and retold, and we can attempt to access these stories through analyses of the things themselves, as biographies. It is context that aids in the creation of narrative for the artefacts and subsequently the settlement and burial sites that are investigated. Understanding that every bead or brooch has entered the archaeological record with an individual biography means that it is possible to look to the context to help understand the potential significance of the item. For example, small bags with assorted contents that can include dress accessories are occasionally found lying around the waist area of female Anglo-Saxon burials. The contents of the bags are not in themselves dress accessories as defined below, but they nevertheless show an attitude towards these ornaments, perhaps indicating an on-going biographical narrative through the practice of curation (Eckardt and Williams 2003, 147) or gift-giving (Kopytoff 1986, 69). The highly varied contents of these bags have also been characterised as amuletic (Meaney 1981, 249–55) or heirlooms (Gilchrist 2012, 237–8) and the latter characterisation can be investigated through the analysis of different generations in cemeteries (e.g. Sayer 2010, 59–91). None of these potential narrative options are mutually exclusive, but they are often neglected in analyses of individual artefact types in favour of immediate meaning or symbolism.

In the seventh to ninth centuries AD, Christianity became the dominant religion of Anglo-Saxon England. Christianity may or may not have impacted immediately on daily practice and identity, and there has been much investigation into the processes of conversion whether identity related, political or otherwise (a range of these approaches is evident in Carver 2003, but also see especially Petts 2011, 36; Urbanczyk 2003). Investigating dress accessories with these different models in mind is one way of accessing a deeper understanding of the changes in expression of worldviews at a micro-level or individual level. This is a time period when burial with dress fittings comes to a potentially abrupt end, as suggested in the recent work on Anglo-Saxon chronology (Bayliss and Hines 2013). Developing a comparative approach within this specific time frame thus offers a chance to develop new ways of approaching dress fittings from non-funerary contexts and provides a means of exploring the effects of religious change on items likely circulating in life before deposition in the grave. Connections between material culture and religious belief or ritual practice are well known (e.g. Meaney 2003, 238; see Gilchrist 2008, 119 for discussion), but there has seldom been any focus on using them to explore ritual actions as part of daily life. 'Mundane' artefacts are now more accepted active elements in the articulation of worldviews (Lucy 1999, 37), but to date dress items have largely been considered in terms of their role within burial assemblages: as datable items and as indicators of dress, fashion and gender (Geake 1997; Crawford 2004) and through their decoration as indicative of certain kinds of belief systems or ideological standpoints (Behr 2000).

This paper considers finds of dress items within cemeteries and settlements. The author takes the view that a separation between rituality and functionality is a false dichotomy in our interpretation of the past (see Brück 1999; Hill 1995). Using a comparative assessment of dress fittings recovered from cemeteries and settlements in Cambridgeshire and Suffolk, it is argued that even when items are single finds, lack extensive decoration or are found without suggestive and interpretable archaeological contexts, such objects can still be explored in terms of having additional meanings or perceptions and that even these apparently simple items may once have had more than a functional role. By comparing the presence of items such as beads, brooches and other personal dress items in graves and their relative presence or absence in settlement contexts it might be possible to suggest that such items may have been intrinsic to the playing out of ritual actions in both life and death.

In this paper dress accessories are defined as personal objects worn on the body primarily for the purposes of decoration, but they may also have had a functional purpose, such as a fastener for clothing. There are of course other items that could fall into this categorisation. A sword, for example, may be worn as both a weapon and as part of warrior or 'military' dress (see Hoss, this volume; Brunning 2013, 143, 241–59). Weapons are not considered here, as although dress accessories such as beads and brooches might have multiple functions or meanings, weapons can be considered to have very specific biographies that need separate consideration, particularly with the array of evidence for their separate votive deposition across historical periods (e.g. Bradley 1998). Secondarily, there is a lack of comparative evidence available from settlement sites. The artefact types considered here fall primarily into the category of adornment and have no obvious immediate secondary function except that of fastening clothing or styling hair (both of which are forms of adornment in themselves, and are actions which have the potential to be imbued with their own significance).

Anglo-Saxon dress accessories in context

The regional study area of Cambridgeshire and Suffolk (boundaries defined by the Historic Environment Records offices as of September 2008) was chosen on the basis of fulfilling several criteria: East Anglia is a key region for large-scale Anglo-Saxon settlement excavations; both counties contain a reasonably large Anglo-Saxon corpus; and this corpus includes a selection of well-published sites as well as a range of grey literature thanks to the implementation of planning guidance (known as PPG16) and developer-funded archaeology since 1990. All the identified sites are excavated settlements that contain phases that fall within the seventh to ninth centuries AD with clearly associated cemeteries, so that any artefacts in the graves can be easily compared to the settlement assemblage. The Conversion/post-Conversion focus allows this study to take place in a period when a known belief system is beginning to take hold in some regions, which can be compared to the archaeological evidence. Many sites are still interpreted in unpublished site reports as likely to be either Christian or containing confusing, seemingly pagan elements, with a distinct lack of understanding surrounding the possibilities of the middle ground in ritual action, or the interaction of these ideologies.

A total of twenty sites with corresponding cemeteries and settlements were identified in the study area (see Fig. 6.1). Dress accessories were found at eight of these sites, although after eliminating those with phasing difficulties or inconsistencies in recording only three contained dress accessories that could be reliably compared in both the settlement and in the burials, (see Tables 6.1 and 6.3). The settlement and cemetery at Bloodmoor Hill, Carlton Colville, Suffolk, contained the widest range of crossover artefacts and as such they form the main case studies for this chapter. Corresponding dress accessories from both settlement and cemetery spheres include pins, beads, pendants, brooches, and lace tags (see Table 6.2). Beads and pendants, however, do not seem to correspond exactly by type: the artefacts are not identical but are of the same general category. A particularly magnificent silver-gilt keystone garnet brooch found in grave 23 is not reflected in the settlement assemblage, but six annular brooches and a further six bow brooches of cruciform and safety pin types were excavated from the settlement. One small fragment of a possible backwards-looking animal type disc-brooch was also identified. It is interesting that such is the rarity of cruciform brooches outside burial contexts (Martin 2015 notes just one of 2075 brooches was found in a stratified context, a sunken-featured building at West Stow), the almost complete one (no. 16) found at Bloodmoor Hill has been suggested to be from an area that might have once been a cemetery with the graves now heavily disturbed and destroyed (Lucy *et al.* 2009, 173). The cruciform brooch itself appears to have been repaired, which is not unusual (Martin 2012, 59–73), but this one has

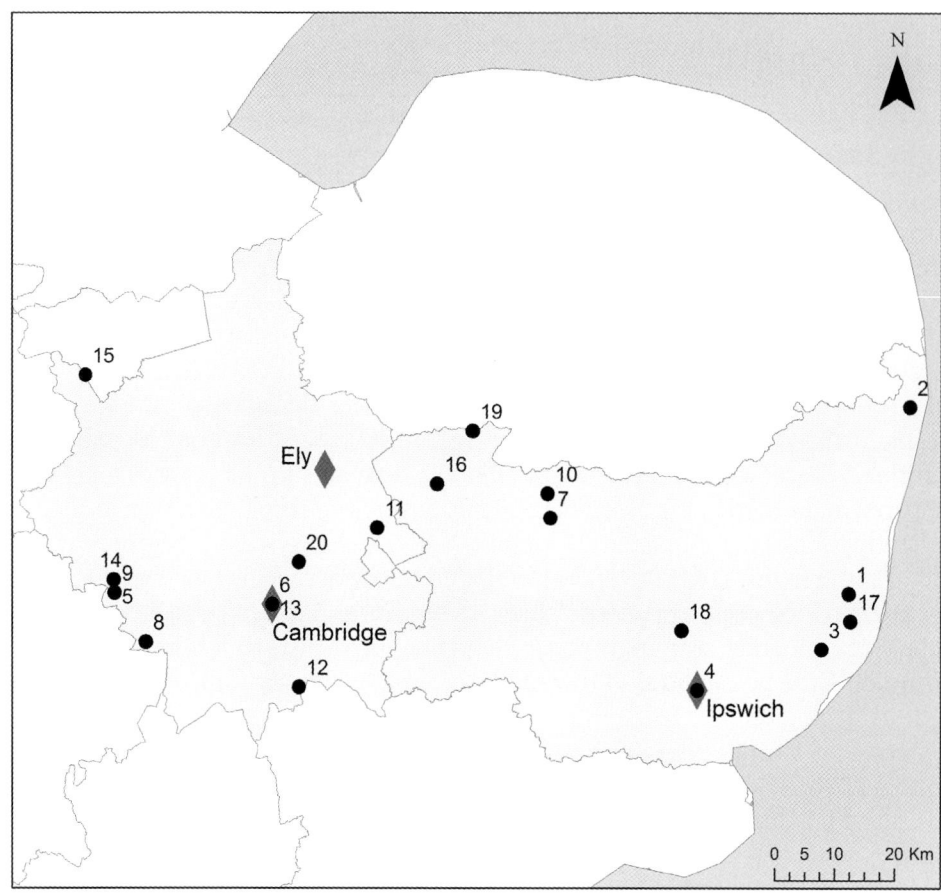

1   Barber's Point, Friston
2   Bloodmoor Hill, Carlton Colville
3   Burrow Hill, Butley
4   Buttermarket and Boss Hall, Ipswich
5   Castle Hills, The Hillings, St. Neots
6   Church End, Cherry Hinton, Cambridge
7   Crows Field, Ixworth Thorpe
8   Station Road, Gamlingay
9   Hall Place, St. Neots
10 Hercules Went, Fakenham Magna
11 Hillside Meadow, Fordham
12 Hinxton Hall, Hinxton
13 Institute of Criminology and Kings Garden Hostel, The Backs, Cambridge
14 Little Paxton Quarry, Little Paxton
15 Minerva Business Park, Alwalton
16 RAF Lakenheath, Eriswell
17 Saint Botolph's Monastery, Iken
18 Smye's Corner, Shrubland Quarry and Vicarage Farm, Coddenham
19 Staunch Meadow/Chequer Meadow, Brandon
20 The Lodge, Waterbeach

Fig. 6.1: Location map of sites included in study area of Cambridgeshire and Suffolk. Diamonds indicate documented Minster sites (map by R. Weetch).

Table 6.1: Sites with dress accessories in either/both the cemetery and settlement areas, and whether the cemetery objects are reflected in the settlement and vice versa

Site	Burials	Settlement	Corresponding artefacts
Bloodmoor Hill	Y	Y	Y
The Backs	Y	Y	N
Burrow Hill	?	Y	N
Brandon	N	Y	N
Coddenham	Y	Y	Y
Gamlingay	N	Y	N
Hillside Meadow	N	Y	N
Church End	N	Y	N
Total with dress accessories	3	8	2

Table 6.2: Dress accessories at Bloodmoor Hill, comparing settlement finds to grave good

Accessory type	Settlement	Cemetery
Beads (all materials)	20	8
Bracelets	3	0
Brooches	12	1
Buckles	8	0
Finger rings	5	0
Girdle hangers/keys	0	3
Hooked tags	2	0
Lace tags	1	3
Pendants	2	11
Pins	54	3
Wrist clasps	4	0

Seven of the 11 cemetery pendants are likely to be from the same necklace in grave 11 (Lucy *et al.* 2009).

not been repaired to the extent that it was fully functional, and hence it has been suggested that it may have been an heirloom or curated item, or at the very least was old when lost or deposited.

Burial has often been interpreted as the area of principal wealth investment simply because the finest artefacts are not so commonly found in settlement contexts. Although it could not be argued that the Bloodmoor Hill burials are among the richest set of known graves, at Bloodmoor Hill silver and gold pendants, the silver-gilt keystone garnet disc brooch, a fine chalcedony bead and the elaborate maplewood casket found in grave 15 all indicate a certain level of finery. The jewellery and dress items from the settlement compare favourably with the grave-goods, and they are not purely indicative of a 'functional' domestic assemblage. Indeed, in some cases the settlement finds almost appear richer than the burials and this is particularly clear for the beads, which include a higher than average proportion of amber examples in comparison to similar settlement sites such as West Stow (Lucy et al. 2009, 176). The five beads found in graves 22 and 13 at Bloodmoor Hill are made of glass and are of plain colours, two red and three green. A further green glass bead was found in grave 15, as well as a chalcedony bead, possibly continental in origin, and a jet/lignite bead in the same grave. In contrast, the twenty beads found in the settlement included considerably more variety, with five polychrome and ten monochrome beads, as well as five amber beads and one of amethyst. It must be noted here that the individual beads found in the Bloodmoor Hill cemetery correspond nicely with the single bead finds from the settlement, which come from a full range of contexts including surface middens, pits, post-holes and the fills of sunken-featured buildings (ibid., 176–9, 394; see Fig. 6.2). Monochrome and polychrome beads both appear as components in necklaces throughout Anglo-Saxon England. However, it is specifically polychrome beads that are more often found in the bag collections mentioned above alongside a range of odd items. The prevalence of various types of beads in the settlement at Bloodmoor Hill could perhaps be seen in the context of these bag collections. Half of the twenty beads from the settlement were monochrome, but the other half of the settlement assemblage is highly varied. Given that Meaney established the prevalence of polychrome and non-glass beads in bag collections (Meaney 1981, 192–210, although she also argued for other bead types including monochrome ones to be considered amuletic), the Bloodmoor Hill bead assemblage is highly suggestive of the use of these purse collections in everyday life.

The amethyst bead is not common in the Anglo-Saxon period, and overall it is more frequent in Kent than East Anglia (Huggett 1988, fig. 2), although it must be said that it is not as rare as Huggett suggests; Geake identifies 90 amethyst beads from 37 graves in her sample of 2583. Other types of amethyst artefact are not present in her review, and neither are there any more amethyst beads from the remaining c. 4417 graves that were not analysed due to poor excavation or publication (Geake 1997, 41). What seems apparent, particularly when we add the identification of amber, jet and organic pendants also present in both the cemetery and the settlement contexts, is that the artefacts found in the settlement are just as 'rich' as those found in the burials, which are mainly present as worn artefacts: 50% of the beads in the settlement were polychrome or non-glass. The major difference is that the beads found in the settlement are single finds with no apparent connection to their use in life, while the beads and pendants in the burials appear mostly to have been suspended from a necklace or connected with silver or copper-alloy wire in bags, with particular combinations of minerals, precious metals and organic material prevalent. Although there is the possibility that later taphonomic processes can account for the instances

6. Middle Anglo-Saxon dress accessories in life and death: expressions of a worldview

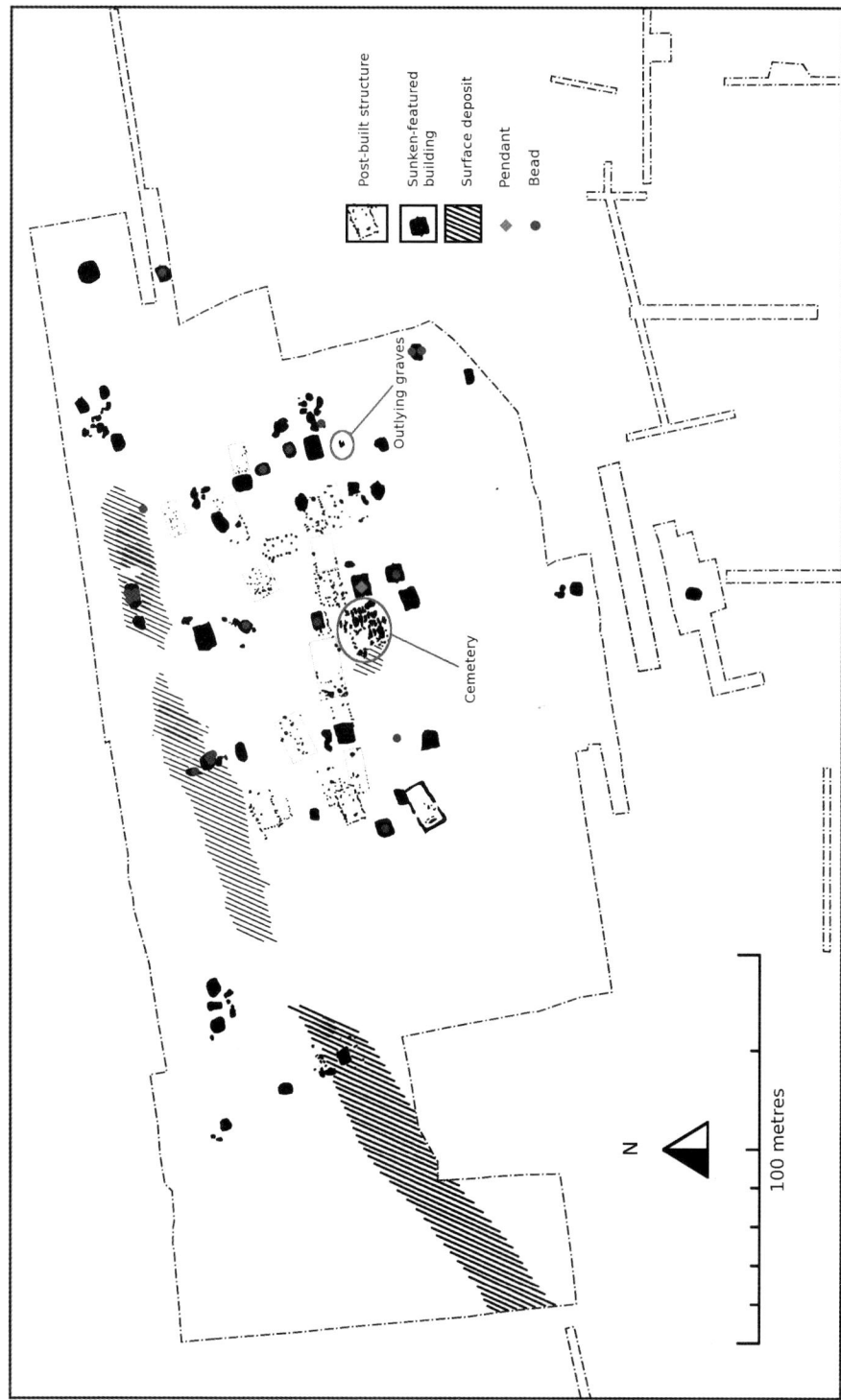

Fig. 6.2: Distribution of beads and pendants at Bloodmoor Hill, Carlton Colville, Suffolk, in all Saxon phases (after Lucy et al. 2009, 39).

Table 6.3: Sites in data set with corresponding cemetery and settlement phasing

Site	Cemetery	Settlement
Bloodmoor Hill	7th century	6th–8th centuries
The Backs	7th century	6th–7th centuries
Burrow Hill	7th–9th centuries (?)	7th–9th centuries
Brandon	8th–9th centuries	7th–9th centuries
Coddenham	7th century	7th century
Gamlingay	9th–10th centuries	6th–10th centuries
Hillside Meadow	8th–9th centuries	6th–12th centuries
Church End	9th–12th centuries	7th–12th centuries

of single beads present in non-cemetery contexts, it is unlikely that disturbance to the cemetery has caused the distribution of the beads in other areas of the site. At Bloodmoor Hill, beads occur in features that pre-date the mid- to late seventh-century cemetery (Lucy *et al.* 2009, 176–9). It is worth noting that the beads from the settlement area at Bloodmoor Hill were mostly found singly rather than together, apart from three amber beads from a sunken-featured building (Structure 17). It is not possible to equate the beads exactly with the amuletic collections Meaney describes (1981, 166–8, 249–53) but this does not necessarily detract from their significance in the settlement sphere as these amuletic collections are varied by their very nature. It is because of their significance within burials and their curation in bag assemblages that we must consider beads found in the settlement sphere to be potentially more than just loss from a broken necklace or falling off an item of clothing it was stitched on to (although these methods of entering the archaeological record and their significance are not mutually exclusive). It can be suggested that the collection or curation of beads from the settlement sphere is part of enchainment, enforcing or creating relations between people and objects (Chapman 2000, 37–9; Fowler 2004, 66), with beads derived from the settlement ('found' objects) placed as collections into graves. It is possible that some of the beads found in graves were once 'found' objects recovered from the settlement by its inhabitants and subsequently worn singly or as parts of necklaces, or even placed in bag collections. In such instances, the bead would connect the buried individual to the settlement and those who inhabited it in the past. Support for such a theory comes from the dating of the beads. Structure 33, a sunken-featured building, contained two beads of 'divergent dates', a fifth- or sixth-century polychrome bead and a seventh- or eighth-century monochrome bead (Lucy *et al.* 2009, 177). If beads were suitable objects for inclusion in a potentially amuletic bag or box assemblage, then their use in the settlement sphere may also be potentially more significant than simply decorative.

Also of particular interest at Bloodmoor Hill are the possible bucket-shaped pendants found in Structure 20 (a sunken-featured building) and the silver anthropomorphic

6. Middle Anglo-Saxon dress accessories in life and death: expressions of a worldview   123

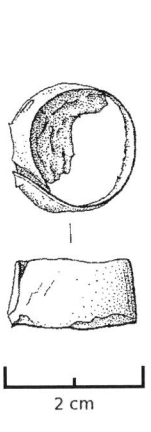
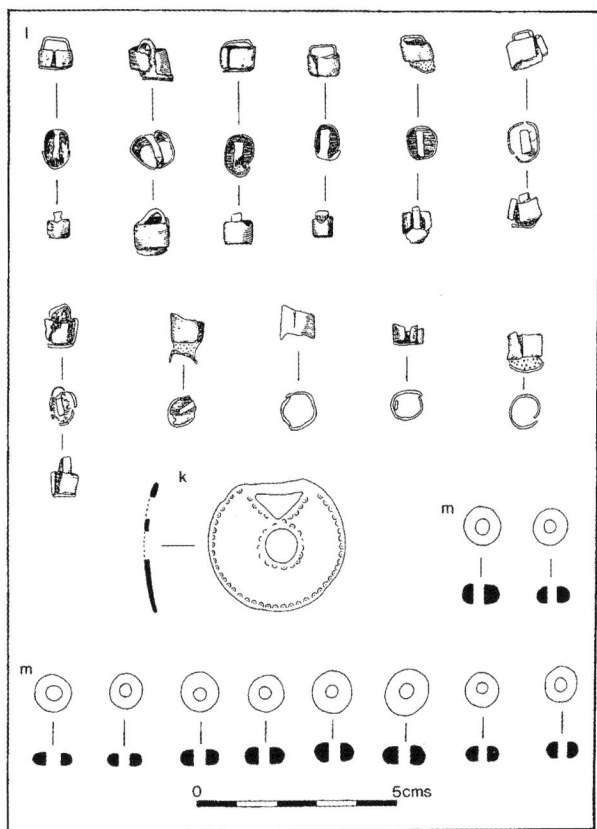

Fig. 6.3: Bucket pendants: left: possible bucket pendant from Bloodmoor Hill (after Lucy et al. 2009, fig. 4.4); right, bucket pendants, a disc pendant and glass beads from Grave HB2 at Bidford-on-Avon (after Dickinson 1993, fig. 6.2).

pendant found unstratified through metal-detection following the excavation (Lucy et al. 2009, 177–8; Fig. 6.3). Both of these pendant types are associated primarily with graves when the provenance is known (Brundle 2013, 203–8), and both are considered to be cultic or amuletic in some way (Webster 2000, 45–6), although Lisa Brundle's analysis suggests anthropomorphic pendants are not necessarily related to burials (Brundle 2013, 214). Audrey Meaney (1981, 219–25) suggested an amuletic significance for amber and jet and indeed organic materials such as wood, bone and animal teeth which are all found incorporated into various types of pendants and collections within Anglo-Saxon graves across England. Meaney may have been rather enthusiastic in her identification of amulets, but the fine example of the probably seventh-century beaver tooth pendant from a grave at Wigber Low, Derbyshire, does suggest special treatment with its setting in a gold mount and introduces the idea of the suspension (as apposed to sewing onto clothing) of amuletic or ideologically significant objects as adornment. This concept is seen in the presence of the silver cross pendant in grave 11 at Bloodmoor Hill, which combines the presence of a pendant within a grave and a known belief system's iconography.

Brundle (2013, 214) indicates that only 12 other similar anthropomorphic figures of the same or similar type are known, none of which exactly parallel this fine example. A similar figure in the British Museum collections (BEP 2001,0711.1) appears to be female, in contrast to the obvious male anatomy of the Bloodmoor Hill example. The rarity of the depiction of the human figure in the early and middle Anglo-Saxon periods is such that this pendant must have been extremely significant, with the use of gesture in the form (*ibid.*, 210–13). The figurine can be included as a dress accessory because it has a suspension loop and was likely to have been worn, although it could also potentially have been strung up somewhere significant. A similar example from the cemetery at Broadstairs in Kent was found hanging from a chatelaine, which potentially links these figurines with bag collections, which were also worn in this way (*ibid.*, 209).

'Bucket-shaped pendants', small copper-alloy objects *c.* 10–20mm wide (sometimes with a looped 'handle'), are also known from Anglo-Saxon graves (see Fig. 6.4), as well as earlier burials on the continent (Dickinson 1993, 50–1), and their function is not well understood. When found in graves there are usually at least two, and sometimes up to twenty, with the possibility that they were sewn onto leather and hung around the neck or placed into a bag or purse hung around the neck (*ibid.*, 51). Traces of textile have sometimes been found inside the bucket-shaped pendants and they are almost exclusively buried with women, although this is not so on the continent (*ibid.*, 51). Tania Dickinson's assessment of an Anglo-Saxon burial with bucket-shaped pendants and a bag assemblage supports the idea that they are in some way amuletic, backing up Audrey Meaney's suggestion of the existence of a female 'cunning woman' in the early Anglo-Saxon period, often associated with a seemingly random selection of items in a bag or sometimes in a box as at Bloodmoor Hill (Dickinson 1993, 45–53; Meaney 1981, 166–8, 249–53).

It is curious, given that formal burial can be considered the result of an expression of a particular belief system, that the presence of such items in the settlement sphere has not been more carefully examined. Anthropomorphic and bucket-shaped pendants are both types of item which may be highly charged, yet are not generally considered to be so when found in a settlement context. That the bucket-shaped pendant was found in a sunken-featured building context is also perhaps interesting, given the potential parallels with burials. Sunken-featured buildings were likely to have been backfilled in one or two episodes, and Hamerow has shown the sunken-featured building to be a particular location for the 'special deposits' she identifies (Hamerow 2006, 8; Sofield 2015). This short episodic backfilling (Tipper 2004, 104–5; Hamerow 2011, 150) could be suggested to parallel the inhumation burial. The presence of such possibly amuletic items within the settlement cannot, therefore, be ignored. Indeed, if we are to understand such objects as amuletic, we must also consider how these items then fit into the conversion to Christianity. Clearly there is a continuing concept of both the use of dress accessories to express worldview (as in the use of pendants, particularly the cross pendant at Bloodmoor Hill, which clearly references a belief system) but it can also be shown through the use of dress accessories that the introduction of Christianity did not diminish the use and ideologies behind those much less Christian-seeming amulets.

Although it is a possibility that the transformative process of the agency of death imbues the ideological significance onto the items placed in graves, there is no reason to suggest that beads or pendants only receive ideological agency on entering the grave, and indeed some evidence to suggest the opposite is true. Items such as the bucket-shaped pendant and the figurine pendant do not have a clearly known function that can readily be identified as something necessary or ordinary to Anglo-Saxon daily life. Thus the presence of such artefacts in settlements – and here we can perhaps add items also present within bag assemblages in graves (including amethyst and amber beads, also present in grave 30 at Coddenham, Suffolk) as similar non-practical objects – indicates something about the settlement itself. Perhaps the artefacts were either present in a ritual action that took place in the lived environment or, on a more simple level, these items may have carried ideological significance when being worn as well as when placed in a grave. The placing of a bead within a bag rather than on a visible necklace or attached visibly to clothing in also indicates the significance held within the item itself rather than its intrinsic appearance. The depositional circumstances of the bucket-shaped pendant in a sunken-featured building with a much later dated safety-pin brooch are also cause for comment, perhaps indicating an element of curation.

In contrast to Bloodmoor Hill, the sites at Coddenham, Suffolk (Everett *et al.* 2003; Penn 2011) and on the Cambridge Backs (Dodwell *et al.* 2004, 95–124) contain fewer artefacts that are reflected in both the grave and the settlement assemblages. Indeed, the excavations on the Backs contain no single item that is represented in both spheres, with the burials containing overtly personal objects: a pin, comb and a copper-alloy Roman bracelet, while the settlement assemblage has no iron items and mainly comprises bulk finds such as pottery, animal bone and fired clay. The site of Coddenham does contain corresponding items, but this is limited to the settlement and the cemetery both containing buckles and knives which are not considered here. Interestingly, the settlement area was selected for excavation due to the high number of metal-detected finds and its proximity to the cemetery across the valley. The finds that are recorded as metal-detected under the Historic Environment Record's entry for Vicarage Farm, Coddenham, correspond much more neatly with the cemetery assemblage, with brooches, buckles, coins, a comb, a knife and a necklace all metal-detected from the settlement area and the object types represented in the cemetery. The metal-detected assemblage is particularly high in gold items, with several thrymsas/tremisses (coins) and fragments of gold dress items, suggesting a very different expression of status to known high-status settlements such as Yeavering or

Lyminge (Thomas and Knox 2012) which simply do not have artefacts of gold, and further stressing the importance of approaching the archaeological record in search of biography and subsequently an individual site narrative – two communities may well have very different attitudes to ornaments and their meanings in life and death, just as their members may have differing levels of wealth in which to purchase and wear these items.

Summary

It is important to move away from using dress accessories as purely regional or 'socio-cultural' markers and towards understanding them as part of a wider culture in which they themselves may have been agents (e.g. in being old or having intangible value placed upon them). The items that Anglo-Saxons chose to adorn their dead may have been their everyday clothes, perhaps their 'special occasion' clothes, or even an outfit specially assembled for the funeral – the fact remains that all of these options represent conscious decisions on the part of those burying the dead. To draw a modern comparison, it is unthinkable to many in the modern western world that a relative might be buried in anything other than a decent set of clothes, even if nobody views the dead. What this does not suggest is that clothing is necessarily ritualised when worn in daily life, but it indicates that there is an attitude and a level of community-wide understanding about the significance of clothing and adornment in life and death. Those more portable objects that are potentially optional such as beads, pendants and brooches (clothing in northwest Europe has to be seen as a necessity in daily life!), may, however, take on a different role with the possibility of a biography of ownership, collection, and decorative motif as well as treatment in life and death all contributing to an agency that may not be as significant in clothing and hairstyles. What the evidence from Bloodmoor Hill and other sites begins to show is that the items selected for inclusion within a burial are clearly referenced in the settlement assemblages, and so do indeed link the two spheres of life and death. While it is difficult, potentially impossible, to suggest what agency these objects actually had, the spheres of life and death are interrelated. Although transformative biographies might be constructed for curated or heirloom items such as beads, pendants or repaired brooches (this last being the cruciform brooch in the Bloodmoor Hill settlement), the significance of these dress accessories in the lived sphere is likely to have affected their inclusion in the sphere of the dead.

It can be suggested that focusing on dress accessories alone as a way of investigating the Anglo-Saxon worldview limits the potential narrative dangerously to using adornment as the primary expression of worldview, belief systems and identity. This is clearly only the case if these items are examined only within funerary contexts. Here the analysis of dress accessories using a broader framework involving the full range of the archaeological record indicates the potential significance of dress accessories in the Anglo-Saxon world, and that it cannot be studied in isolation. It is not possible to get to an exact meaning or conclusion regarding a particular ritual action, but acknowledging that these actions and meanings are possible goes a long way to expanding our comprehension of the complexity of the Anglo-Saxon worldview in the seventh to ninth centuries AD and allows space for the interpretation of the process of conversion to Christianity. It is because of the inclusion of dress accessories within graves and in bag and box assemblages, and the ubiquity of such personal items that may have both their own biography and direct links to the biographies of individuals or ancestors, that dress accessories in context can be understood as more than decorative and symbolic. They are an intricate and inextricable part of the everyday experience of Anglo-Saxon peoples and their worldview, and approaching dress accessories in this way in any period in the past where such items are present in the spheres of the dead and the living has great potential to enlighten our understanding of such inaccessible regions of the past as worldviews and beliefs.

Acknowledgements

This chapter comes out of my doctoral research completed in 2012 at the University of Reading. I would like to thank my supervisors Roberta Gilchrist and Gabor Thomas for their expert supervision and my examiners Grenville Astill and Andrew Reynolds, for their helpful suggestions and guidance. I particularly thank the anonymous reviewers who provided excellent guidance and suggested many improvements to this paper. I could not have completed my research without the expert advice and time from the staff at the Cambridgeshire and Suffolk HERs and Suffolk County Council Archaeological Services.

Bibliography

Bayliss, A. and Hines, J., eds. (2013) *Anglo-Saxon Graves and Grave Goods of the 6th and 7th Centuries AD: A Chronological Framework.* London, Society for Medieval Archaeology.
Behr, C. (2000) The origins of kingship in early medieval Kent. *Early Medieval Europe* 9, 25–52.
Bradley, R. (1998) *The Passage of Arms: an Archaeological Analysis of Prehistoric Hoards and Votive Deposits.* Oxford, Oxbow Books.
Brück, J. (1999) Ritual and rationality: some problems of interpretation in European archaeology. *European Journal of Archaeology* 2, 313–44.
Brundle, L. (2013) The body on display: exploring the role and use of figurines in early Anglo-Saxon England. *Journal of Social Archaeology* 13, 197–219.
Brunning, S. (2013) *The 'Living' Sword in Early Medieval Northern Europe: an Interdisciplinary Study.* Unpublishd PhD thesis, University College London.
Carver, M. (2003) *The Cross Goes North: Processes of Conversion in Northern Europe, AD 300–1300.* York/Woodbridge, York Medieval Press in association with Boydell & Brewer.
Chapman, J. L. (2000) *Fragmentation in Archaeology: People, Places and Broken Objects in the Prehistory of South-Eastern Europe.* London, Routledge.
Crawford, S. (2004) Votive deposition, religion and the Anglo-Saxon furnished burial ritual. *World Archaeology* 36, 87–102.

Dickinson, T. (1993) An Anglo-Saxon 'cunning woman' from Bidford-on-Avon. In M. Carver (ed.) *In Search of Cult: Archaeological Excavations in Honour of Philip Rahtz*. Woodbridge, Boydell Press.
Dodwell, N., Lucy, S. and Tipper, J. (2004) Anglo-Saxons on the Cambridge Backs: the Criminology site settlement and King's Garden Hostel cemetery. *Proceedings of the Cambridge Antiquarian Society* 93, 95–124.
Eckardt, H. and Williams, H. (2003) Objects without a past? The use of Roman objects in early Anglo-Saxon graves. In H. Williams (ed.) *Archaeologies of Remembrance: Death and Memory in Past Societies*, 141–70. New York and London, Kluwer/Plenum.
Everett, L., Anderson, S., Powell, K and Riddler, I. (2003) *Archaeological Evaluation Report: Vicarage Farm, Coddenham. CDD 022. An Archaeological Evaluation, 2003.* Ipswich, Suffolk County Council Archaeological Service.
Fisher, G and Loren, D. D. (2003) Introduction: embodying identity in archaeology. *Cambridge Archaeological Journal* 13(2), 225–30.
Fowler, C. (2004) *The Archaeology of Personhood: an Anthropological Approach*. London, Routledge.
Geake, H. (1997) *The Use of Grave-Goods in Conversion-Period England c. 600–c. 850*. Oxford, John and Erica Hedges (British Archaeological Reports, British Series 261).
Gell, A. (1998) *Art and Agency: an Anthropological Theory*. Oxford, Clarendon.
Gilchrist, R. (2012) *Medieval Lives: Archaeology and the Life Course*. Woodbridge, Boydell and Brewer.
Gilchrist, R. (2008) Magic for the dead? The archaeology of magic in later medieval burials. *Medieval Archaeology* 52, 119–59.
Hamerow, H. (2006) 'Special Deposits' in Anglo-Saxon Settlements. *Medieval Archaeology* 50, 1–30.
Hamerow, H. (2011) Anglo-Saxon timber buildings and their social context. In H. Hamerow, D. A. Hinton and S. Crawford (eds.) *The Oxford Handbook of Anglo-Saxon Archaeology*, 128–55. Oxford, Oxford University Press.
Hill, J. D. (1995) *Ritual and Rubbish in the Iron Age of Wessex: a Study on the Formation of a Specific Archaeological Record*. Oxford, Tempus Reparatum (British Archaeological Reports, British Series 242).
Hodder, I. (2011) Human-thing entanglement: towards an integrated archaeological perspective. *Journal of the Royal Anthropological Institute* 17, 154–77.
Huggett, J. W. (1988) Imported grave goods and the early Anglo-Saxon economy. *Medieval Archaeology* 32, 63–96.
Keefer, S. L., Jolly, K. L. and Karkov, C. E. (2010) *Cross and Cruciform in the Anglo-Saxon World: Studies to Honor the Memory of Timothy Reuter.* Morgantown, West Virginia University Press.
Kopytoff, I. (1986) The cultural biography of things: commoditization as process. In A. Appadurai (ed.) *The Social Life of Things: Commodities in Cultural Perspective*, 64–91. Cambridge, Cambridge University Press.
Lucy, S. J. (1999) The early Anglo-Saxon burial rite: moving towards a contextual understanding. In M. Rundkvist (ed.) *Grave matters: Eight Studies of First Millennium AD Burials in Crimea, England and Southern Scandinavia: papers from a session held at the European Association of Archaeologists Fourth Annual Meeting in Göteborg 1998*, 33–40. Oxford, Archaeopress (British Archaeological Reports, International Series 781).
Lucy, S., Tipper, J. and Dickins, A. (2009) *The Anglo-Saxon settlement and cemetery at Bloodmoor Hill, Carlton Colville, Suffolk*. Cambridge, Cambridge Archaeological Unit.
Martin, T. F. (2012) Riveting biographies. The theoretical implications of early Anglo-Saxon brooch repair, customisation and use-adaptation. In B. Jervis and A. Kyle (eds.) *Make Do and Mend: The Archaeology of Compromise?* 59–73. Oxford, Archaeopress (British Archaeological Reports, International Series 2408).
Martin, T. F. (2014) (Ad)Dressing the Anglo-Saxon body: corporeal meanings and artefacts in early England. In P. Blinkhorn and C. Cumberpatch (eds.), *The Chiming of Crack'd Bells: Recent Approaches*

to the Study of Artefacts in Archaeology, 27–38. Oxford, Archaeopress (British Archaeological Reports, International Series 2677).

Martin, T. F. (2015) *The Cruciform Brooch and Anglo-Saxon England*. Woodbridge, Boydell and Brewer.

Mauss, M. (1973) Techniques of the body. *Economy and Society* 2, 70–88.

Meaney, A. (1981) *Anglo-Saxon Amulets and Curing Stones*. Oxford, British Archaeological Reports (British Archaeological Reports, British Series 96).

Meaney, A. (2003) Anglo-Saxon pagan and early Christian attitudes to the dead. In M. Carver (ed.) *The Cross Goes North: Processes of Conversion in Northern Europe, AD 300-1300*, 229–42. York, York Medieval Press.

Parker Pearson, M. (1999) *The Archaeology of Death and Burial*. Stroud, Sutton.

Penn, K. (2011) *The Anglo-Saxon cemetery at Shrubland Hall Quarry, Coddenham, Suffolk*. Bury St Edmunds, Suffolk County Council Archaeological Service in conjunction with ALGAO East (East Anglian Archaeology Report 139).

Petts, D. (2011) *Pagan and Christian: Religious Change in Early Medieval Europe*. London, Bristol Classical Press.

Sayer, D. (2010) Death and the family. *Journal of Social Archaeology* 10, 59–91.

Sofield, C. (2015) Anglo-Saxon placed deposits before and during Christianization (5th–9th c.). *Neue Studien zur Sachsenforschung* 5, 111–20.

Thomas, G. and Knox, A. (2012) A window on Christianisation: transformation at Anglo-Saxon Lyminge, Kent, England. *Antiquity* (project gallery). Webpage available at: www.antiquity.ac.uk/projgall/thomas334/ [accessed March 2016].

Tilley, C. (2006) Objectification. In C. Tilley, W. Keane, S. Kuechler-Fogden, M. Rowlands and P. Spyer (eds.) *Handbook of Material Culture*: 60–73. London, Sage.

Tipper, J. (2004) *The Grubenhaus in Anglo-Saxon England: an Analysis and Interpretation of the Evidence from a Most Distinctive Building Type*. Yedingham, Landscape Research Centre.

Urbanczyk, P. (2003) The politics of conversion in North Central Europe. In M. Carver (ed.) *The Cross Goes North: Processes of Conversion in Northern Europe, AD 300-1300*. York/Woodbridge, York Medieval Press in association with Boydell & Brewer.

Webster, L. (2000) Carlton Colville, Suffolk: Anglo-Saxon part-gilded silver pendant figure (M&ME 211). *Treasure Annual Report 2000*, 45–6.

Weetch, R. (2014) *Brooches in Late Anglo-Saxon England within a North West European Context. A Study of Social Identities between the Eighth and Eleventh Centuries*. Unpublished PhD Thesis, Department of Archaeology, University of Reading.

Chapter 7

'Best' gowns, kerchiefs and pantofles: gifts of apparel in the north-east of England in the sixteenth century

Eleanor R. Standley

Introduction

The moveable goods under consideration in this chapter are clothes and accessories bequeathed to family and friends by testators in the north-east of England in the sixteenth century. The sources investigated are a selection of wills and probate inventories proved by the registrars of the bishops of Durham between *c*. 1500 and 1580, and written by merchants, squires, knights, husbandmen, shopkeepers, widows, smiths, saddlers, and cooks, among others. Despite the biases inherent in the documents, the discussion presented below reveals their value in investigating dress when combined with the comparatively sparse archaeological evidence of sixteenth-century clothing, textiles and leather.

In this chapter the scant organic evidence of dress from archaeology is reviewed, followed by some of the studies that have used documents in the examination of early modern dress. Next, the potential of the evidence to inform and expand our knowledge of dress in the sixteenth century is highlighted with respect to articles of clothing found in the north-east wills and inventories. Finally, the significance of gift-giving and memory concerning specific items of clothing is presented. This chapter is intended to introduce the wide variety of evidence and its importance in our understanding of dress in combination with archaeological material, without dwelling on the single identity of an individual or group, or people's obedience of sumptuary legislation.

The wills examined are from those published in Raine's 1835 volume, which contains transcriptions of 323 wills dated from the eleventh century to 1580. Individual wills and inventories are referred to by their number in the publication, with a prefix of R.1835. The north-east region has both surviving wills and inventories with transcriptions, and archaeological dress finds from excavations that can be synthesised and compared. The area was nationally and internationally important, and Newcastle-upon-Tyne was a centre for the diffusion of social, cultural and religious ideas. In 1334 it was the fourth richest town in England, and by the early seventeenth century it was 'fully part of the burgeoning mercantile economy of Europe' (Graves and Heslop 2013, 2). Despite this, the north-east has a low profile in archaeological literature nationally, long seen as 'peripheral' (Petts with Gerrard 2006, 219). The excavated post-medieval evidence of the region has potential to expand our knowledge by the exploration of social and thematic matters of the later- to post-medieval transition (Petts with Gerrard 2006; Standley 2013; Graves and Heslop 2013).

In the last 20 years archaeological objects, such as dress fasteners, fittings, and finger rings, and archaeological theoretical approaches have enhanced our knowledge of early modern dress, and that of the vernacular. Dress accessory small finds are ubiquitous in later medieval and post-medieval sites in Britain. The database of the Portable Antiquities Scheme (PAS) is ever increasing with records of such chance finds; and studies on early modern dress accessories are developing (Egan and Forsyth 1997; Gaimster *et al.* 2002; Standley 2013). However, medieval and early modern clothing and textiles rarely survive in the archaeological record. When they do, the type of deposit they are preserved in biases the textiles that can survive; for example, anaerobic, acidic conditions are particularly detrimental to linen, and humic soils lead to staining of cloths (Crowfoot *et al.* 2001, 2). Furs are absent from excavations, and buried leather can only survive in anaerobic conditions. Excavations on waterlogged sites in London have recovered well over a thousand pieces of footwear including pattens of leather and wood, and hundreds of textile fragments (Grew and de Neergaard 2001; Egan 2005, 17–32, 58–61; Crowfoot *et al.* 2001). Southampton, Winchester and York have yielded textile and footwear evidence, and other medieval sites have produced small fragments of textiles which are often analysed for their weave and dyes (Crowfoot 1975; Walton Rogers 2011; Platt and Coleman-Smith 1975; Crowfoot 1990; Walton Rogers 1997; Bennett with Muthesius 1987; Bennett 1982; Ryder and Gabra-Sanders 1992; Andersson Strand *et al.* 2010). Clothing and shoes found hidden in buildings can be added to the archaeological evidence. Although cases of fifteenth- and sixteenth-century textiles are rare, the practice dates back to at least the early fourteenth century and continued through to the early twentieth century (Swann 1996; Eastop 2006; Deliberately Concealed Garments Project).

The wreck of the *Mary Rose*, which sank in 1545, is an exceptional source that has provided archaeologists with the largest collection of clothing and footwear from a secure context anywhere in the United Kingdom with many of the 655 items associated with skeletal remains (Forster *et al.* 2005, 18). This collection includes a wide range of material from the different social levels present on the ship, from the officers to the ordinary sailors and soldiers. With 257 pieces of footwear, including 70 pairs of shoes and boots, a diversity of styles and designs are represented (*ibid.*). Despite the wide social spectrum however, the evidence is limited to predominantly leather and wool, and are all male items of clothing.

In the north-east, excavations in Newcastle's Castle Ditch at the Black Gate uncovered textile fragments, leather pieces from cobblers, and domestic cast-offs in a series of dumped rubbish contexts (Vaughan 1981, 184–90; Walton 1981, 190–228). These finds form a tangible link to some of the types of early and mid-sixteenth-century textiles and accessories worn in the region. Woollens represent the majority of the textile finds: 443 of the 496 fragments; whereas the vegetable fibres of linen did not survive well in the wet conditions (Walton 1981, 190, 201). While the finds point to manufacturing techniques, and can highlight imports and trade, they provide no evidence of the whole, finished garment, nor of the owners and how the articles were used in daily life.

The archaeological evidence of the textiles and leather of sixteenth century dress is therefore limited, in terms of both quantity and quality. This article does not routinely describe the evidence (archaeological or textual) but combines the material to understand people and their everyday clothing, using the north-east as a case study area. The documents, archaeological material culture and theoretical ideas of phenomenology, consumption, gift-giving, memory, and identities are used to create a more meaningful historical archaeology (see Gilchrist 2009), with a focus on what Bailey (2007, 201) describes as 'individual agency, inter-personal interactions and perception'.

Documentary sources and dress

Wills and probate inventories are a source of evidence that can be successfully interrogated in archaeological studies, as demonstrated by Standley (2013) and Heley (2009). The gifts in the wills were legal bequests for the disposition of the personal estate after the death of the testator. The bequests handed down to family members or friends can provide information about what was owned and worn, and the significance they held to the original owner and the receiver. Wills and inventories have more often been a focus of seventeenth- and eighteenth-century studies in the discipline of history, especially when investigating consumption and large-scale social transformations (Weatherill 1988; 1993; McKendrick et al. 1983; Overton et al. 2004). The later medieval religious aspects of charitable gifts and the provision for the health of the soul are also themes investigated by historians (Burgess 1987), as are financial and legal features, and the different roles of men and women and the material that they bequeathed (for example see Arkell et al. 2000; Spufford 2000a; Erikson 2002; Overton et al. 2004; Biggs 2007).

A major criticism of using wills as an historical source is that they are overly representative of the affluent and male testators. However, the presence of the poor *is* seen in wills when they are the recipients of bequests, and wealth was not the only factor used to decide whether to create a formal will or not (Heley 2009, 10; Issa 1988, 292). The lack of wills made by wives does create a vacuum of evidence as married women were not legally allowed to make a will without the permission of their husbands, therefore, most legal female testators were unmarried or widows (see Erikson 2002 and Biggs 2007). Any missing evidence or gaps that have been criticised in historical studies should not invalidate what *is* recorded, as Heley (2009, 16) argues. In archaeology, it is the nature of the discipline that there are lacunae in the evidence, and that other sources, such as the wills and inventories, and new methods of enquiry are required to further our understanding of possessions and life in the past.

In the last 20 years an interest in clothing of the past and dress history has featured a great deal in studies of the later medieval and early modern periods, especially of the latter. Rosenthal (2009) provides an overview of studies of 'cultures of clothing' and histories of dress up to 2009. The piece, mainly relying on Italian evidence and that of the early modern period, illustrates that on the whole studies are still often concentrated on consumption and the value of clothes; production, retail and shopping; group identities; and the distinction between fashion, clothing, dress and costume. The author does not refer to archaeological research, but does highlight 'the complex field of inquiry that bridges a wide range of scholarly disciplines and methodologies' and that future 'cross-cultural, interdisciplinary studies' are required as no one scholar has the skills or access to material needed to fully answer questions about the history of dress (*ibid.*, 475–6). These are important points to remember, as is the need to recognise that the evidence, be it preserved costumes in museums, documents, or excavated material, adds to our understanding, and that approaches from many disciplines can contribute to the investigation of dress, rather than fully answer any one question.

Many historical studies that use documentary evidence to investigate aspects of dress in the later medieval and early modern periods may be referred to. Hayward, for example, has written extensively on dress, and in *Rich Apparel* (2009) the quantitative analysis of early Tudor wills revealed how often different garments were bequeathed by male and female testators in different social groups in Henrician England. The investigation placed the apparel into the wider context of the law and sumptuary legislation at the time, and how one's wardrobe was used for display and definition of one's place in society (*ibid.*). The value of wills in discussing clothing in early Tudor England is made evident. In a similar vein, Burkholder (2005) examined amounts of household textiles and apparel in relation to the status and sex of will makers, and sumptuary legislation, in her study of wills from the fourteenth and fifteenth centuries. As with Hayward (2009), the evidence from wills was predominantly used to investigate the material evidence of identities (gender and status) and the sumptuary laws, rather than the garments themselves or the agency behind the bequests. Nevertheless, the study highlighted what a surprising amount of information on later medieval clothing and household textiles could be drawn from a relatively few wills that was otherwise irrecoverable (Burkholder 2005, 153).

The consumption of second-hand objects and clothing and its economic significance is one that has been a key feature in post-medieval studies. Margaret Spufford (1976; 1984) has researched documentary evidence to examine early modern non-elites, for example, chapmen. A later publication also used the fragmented documentary evidence to investigate the cost of apparel in seventeenth-century England, demonstrating that probate accounts (rather than wills or probate inventories) can add to our knowledge of clothing worn by 'non-noble, non-gentle groups in society' (Spufford 2000b, 678). Again, this work examined the economic value and separate prices of different garments, and applied a statistical approach. Spufford (2000b, 685) herself recognised that:

> 'The temptation of itemized lists of this type [probate accounts] ... is to produce at least elementary statistics that will give the reader an idea of the "normal" as against the "exceptional", which may have been stumbled on by mistake. The inevitable problem, though, is that once the historian has viable statistics and adequate samples, he or she also tends to lose all sense of individual people.'

As Spufford (*ibid.*) has highlighted the problem of statistical analysis, this chapter will avoid a quantitative approach, and will deal with the individual people and articles of clothing. Perhaps this will predispose the discussion to the 'exceptional' to a certain extent, but there is neither the scope nor desire here to perform statistics on the data and lose the individuals.

A final study worth noting is Tankard's (2012) examination of legal depositions and clothing of the rural poor in seventeenth-century Sussex. She argued that wills and inventories give only a '*static* view of clothing ... the finished, and inert, garment, with no indication of how it was produced or acquired or how it was worn,' whereas the depositions reveal a '*dynamic* view of clothing – including its production, acquisition and appearance, either on or off the body' (*ibid.*, 7). Archaeological dress accessory finds can be 'dynamic' in terms of their significance to their owners and how they can illuminate past lives (Standley 2013), and so too can evidence from inventories and wills give the 'dynamic' view, especially when combined with archaeological evidence and approaches.

The north-east apparel

The north-east wills and inventories acquaint us with the clothes people owned and create a vivid image of the materials used, from furs, to colourful taffetas and velvets. Items seldom mentioned in archaeological literature, such as slippers or satin nightcaps are also found. The documents provide evidence of the material used to produce the clothing and its appearance; shopping and retail information, including valuations; when the apparel was worn; who inherited articles and additional information about the clothes' life histories; and clothes' function as heirlooms and perhaps their emotional and symbolic worth.

A rich array of apparel is revealed in the wills and probate inventories. Gowns, cloaks, kirtles, breeches, hose, stomachers, petticoats, doublets, jerkins, kerchiefs, and coats are some of the garments, along with accessories, including hats, caps, shoes, boots, slippers, girdles, rosaries, rings, chains, brooches, and buttons.

Materials, colours and decorative features are used to describe and identify them in the documents. The examination in this section presents a selection of the apparel and individual owners to widen our interpretation and archaeological enquiry into key elements of dress. For example, privately worn items are usually invisible in the archaeological record and rarely depicted in artworks, so can the wills shed light on clothes like undergarments or nightwear? The identification of 'best' items has usually been read as a measure of quantity (and quality), but we can discover more about 'best' items, and ask are best clothes those worn on the holy day? Particular types of clothing, such as headgear, gloves and footwear can also be explored.

While the excavated contemporary leather footwear from Castle Ditch, Newcastle, is relatively meagre in number and fragmentary in nature, their discussion can be enhanced by the belongings chosen as bequests and listed in inventories. A jerkin maker's inventory details footwear, and indicates that someone specialising in the manufacture of one type of garment – jerkins – was not limited to selling them alone. The 1569 shop inventory of Thomas Johnes, a jerkin maker in Gateshead, included eight made jerkins (Fig. 7.1); a pair of sleeves; calf, goat and kid skins; and three yards of yellow cotton.[1] But he also had one pair of buskin legs (buskins were calf or knee high leather boots), two pair of buskins (iijs), six pairs of 'pantobles' [pantofles] (overshoes with a vamp and deep cork sole, but no quarters) and one pair of 'pompes' [pumps] which were a light, heelless shoe held onto the foot only by their close fit. The total value for all seven pairs was vj^s.vj^d. 'Pumps and pantofles' can be found referred to together in literature suggesting they were worn as a set (see John Florio's *First Fruites*, 1578, f.2v), hence why Thomas would have been selling the two items in his shop. An extant pantofle, but missing its cork sole (Fig. 7.2), has been excavated from Newcastle Castle Ditch from the early sixteenth-century phase of dumping from a cobbler, and a pair is depicted being worn by Elizabeth, Countess of Worcester, on her effigy in Chepstow, dated 1549 (Vaughan 1981, 184–5; no. 510).

Excavated material from the same phase of dumped cobbler's waste included a boot upper (Vaughan 1981, 186, no. 513), which may have been similar to leather pieces

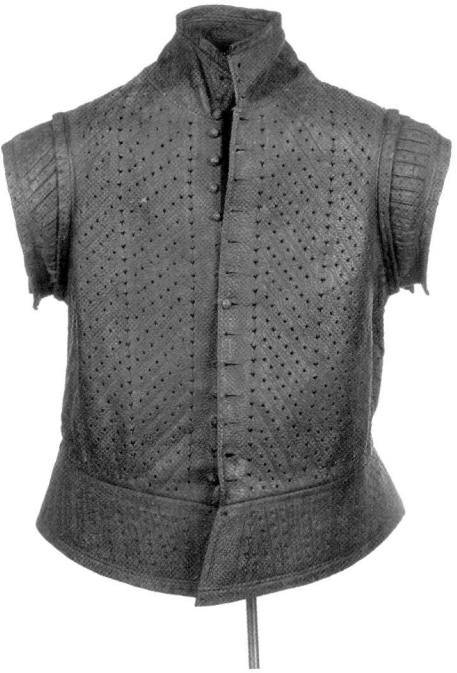

Fig. 7.1: A youth's decorative dark brown leather jerkin decorated with pinking and pewter buttons, dating from the second half of the sixteenth century in the Museum of London collection (36.237; height 520mm; width (shoulders) 450mm) (©Museum of London).

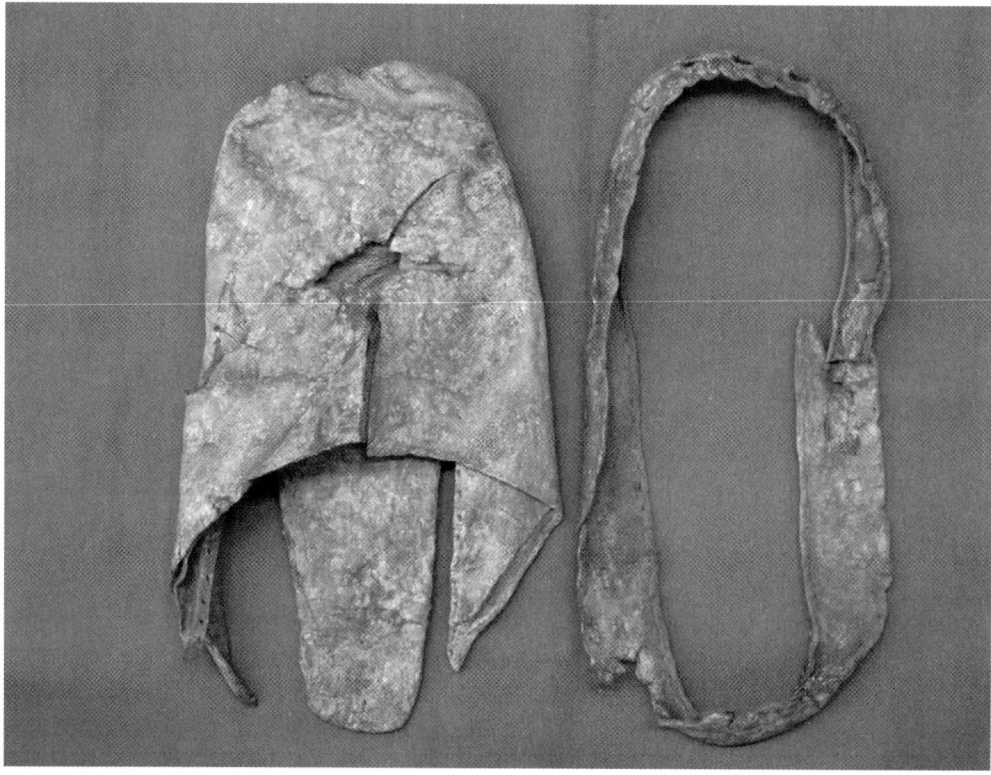

Fig. 7.2: Remains of the leather pantofle from the Castle Ditch dump at the Black Gate, Newcastle-upon-Tyne, lined with goatskin, but missing its cork sole. Vamp and insole (left), and sole cover (right). Insole length 21.5cm. Great North Museum, Newcastle (photograph Jenny Vaughan).

that made up the buskins Thomas was selling. The goatskins in Thomas' shop may have been used for footwear, not just the jerkins, as the upper of the pantofle from Castle Ditch was lined with goatskin (*ibid.*, no. 510). Thomas also had a pair of lasts in his shop. Some of the other shoes bequeathed and inventoried in the early to mid-sixteenth century may have been fashionable 'eared' shoes; a fragment of an eared insole was found in the Castle Ditch (dumping phase *c.* 1525–1550) and a whole shoe of this style was recovered from the *Mary Rose* (*ibid.*, no. 516; Forster *et al.* 2005, fig. 2.45). Only fragments of leather shoes were recovered from the Castle Ditch, but from the documents we learn of the other types and materials of footwear available, such as velvet shoes and velvet slippers.[2]

Velvet was used for many items other than shoes: caps, hats, religious vestments, doublets, breeches, jackets, gowns, jerkins, nightcaps, straight caps, purses, sleeves and edgings. Silk clothing and accessories are also relatively common in the documents. References to silk hats, points, laces, sleeves, stomachers, purses, gowns, ribbons, belts, buttons, doublets, decorative features on petticoats, and other household furnishings can be found. In the inventory of single woman Margaret Gascgoine, dated 1567, a gown and kirtle of 'changeable taffeta' are listed.³ This silk material was described as such because it had a changing colour effect due to a different coloured warp and weft (also known as shot silk). Together with changeable taffeta garments, Margaret owned a gown and kirtle made of silk grogram. The gowns were described as being decorated with silk lace – the changeable taffeta's decoration was gold lace and it was worth the substantial sum of lxvj^s viij^d. 'Changeable' taffeta is referred to in Shakespeare's *Twelfth Night* (2:iv), where Duke Orsino is told that his tailor should make his doublet out of changeable taffeta to reflect his changing, 'opal' mind. A contemporary audience would have been familiar with the fabric and the metaphor. The fabric is cleverly depicted in Hans Holbein the Younger's miniature portrait of Henry Brandon (Fig. 7.3). Despite not knowing the colours of Margaret Gascgoine's taffeta, the luxurious changeable gown, decorated with gold lace must have been opulent and eye catching.

In merchant John Wilkinson's detailed inventory at least 11 different silks were referred to, including coal black silk, skenes of silk, raw silk, silk seams, green raw silk, crimson in grain silk, and 'all colour of sewing silk'.⁴ These tally with the archaeological evidence from later medieval London which suggests that silk thread was used for seams and hems on woven silk and on woollen cloth, and for strengthening button holes and eyelets, securing buttons, decorative topstitching, and decorative braids and edges (Crowfoot *et al.* 2001, 152). Three definite silk fragments were excavated from Castle Ditch, plus other possible pieces. Commenting upon this, Walton (1981, 201) states that 'The small proportion of silk to wool [excavated] is a reflection of the comparative availability of these fabrics at the time'. However, Wilkinson in 1571 was stocked with an array of silks and Margaret Gasgoine had access to enough shot silk to have a gown and kirtle made. In a shop in Bishop Auckland, John Bayles stocked a vast six gross of silk buttons, 7oz of oxen silk, 3oz of coloured silk, ribbon of silk, black sewing silk, along with cloth, other accessories, soap and spices.⁵ This evidence suggests that the small proportion of silk in the dumped rubbish of Castle Ditch reflects, not the availability, but the value of the material to tailors and owners. Clever tailoring would have reused odd shaped scraps of silk, perhaps as buttons or edging, rather than throwing them out.

Taffeta and silk were used for making hats as well. Other forms of the accessory were bonnets, under caps, priest's caps, square caps and straight caps. Robert Lord Ogle of Bothal, in 1562, identified one of his caps by its decoration: 'I gyve to Sr Rob'rt Vghtryd Knight my best velvet gowne and my capp wth aglets and a broche vpon ytt'.⁶ Aglets of gold were worn in pairs and were decorative features on clothing and hats in the sixteenth century. In many portraits, paired aglets decorating hats can be seen, such as in Figure 7.3, and Hans Holbein the Younger's *William Parr, later Marquess of Northampton*, (*c*. 1538–42, The Royal Collection, RCIN 912231). Two fine gold examples of aglets have been found in London and the Wing area (Buckinghamshire) both recorded on the PAS (see Awais-Dean this volume, Fig 8.1; 2011T44/LON-F2F3A4;

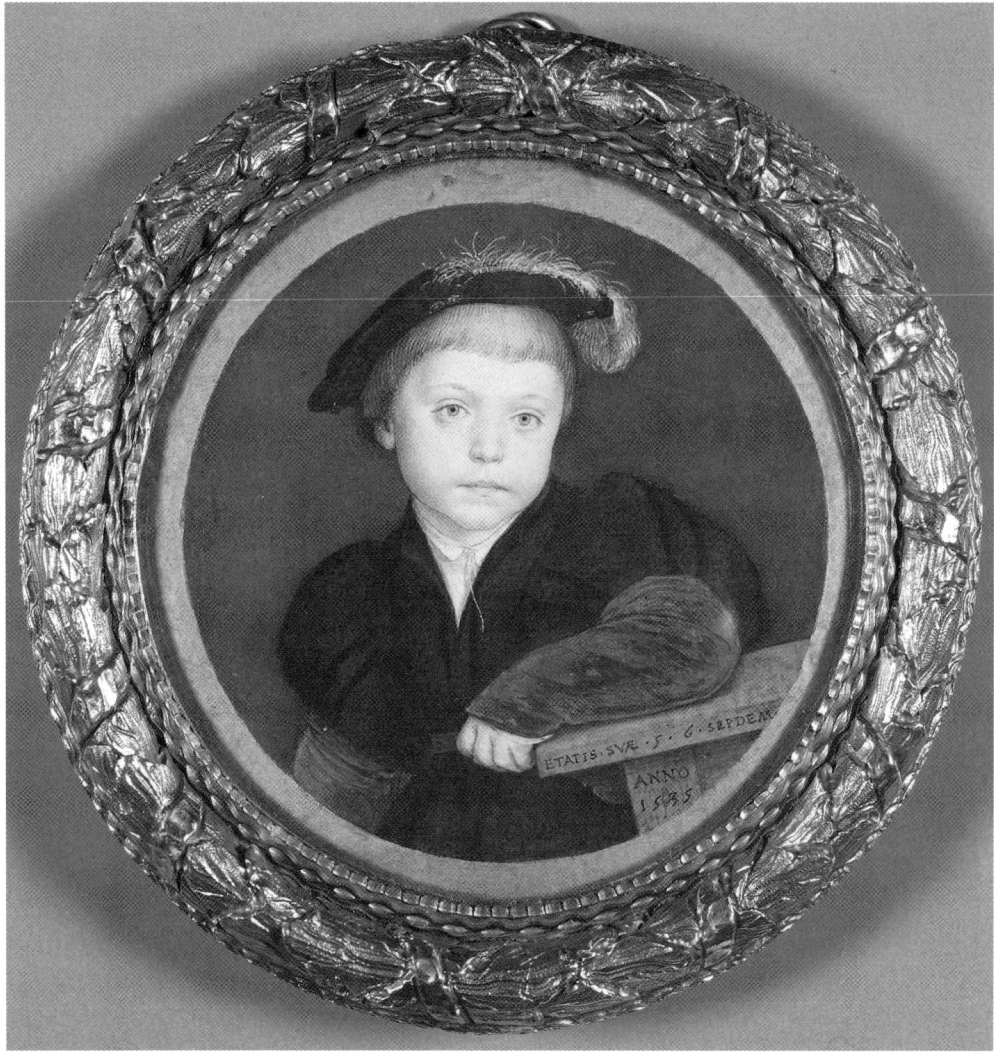

Fig. 7.3: The miniature portrait of Henry Brandon, 2nd Duke of Suffolk, by Hans Holbein the Younger, c. 1541. The sleeves of his doublet are depicted in the luxurious changeable taffeta of peacock green and red. His hat is decorated with pairs of gold aglets. RCIN 422294 Royal Collection Trust (©Her Majesty Queen Elizabeth II 2016).

2011T854/BUCE33633). Other hat decoration could have been buttons, as a cap of Bertram Anderson is described as 'one buttoned cap xij^s'.

Hat or cap badges too have been recorded on the PAS, for example, the silver badges decorated with religious and secular figures and motifs (for example 2014T523/BUC-3409BD, 2012T9281/NCL-9D6371; SWYOR-0E13B5; ESS-D91287 and YORYM-A6C928). The badge that decorated Lord Ogle's cap may have been decorated with a devotional scene, or with a secular motif derived from the Ogle family coat of arms. The will of Sir John Delaval, of Seaton Delaval, High Sherriff of Northumberland, also refers to a brooch worn upon his velvet cap, but it is the brooch rather than the hat which is the gift; 'I gyue to Anne Rames my best broche that is vpon my velvett Capp'.[7] It is interesting to note that the best brooch owned by Sir Delaval was worn on a piece of headgear, rather than a doublet or cloak; the cap could have been worn with any outfit and there would have been no need to reattach the brooch to different pieces in his wardrobe.

The archaeological evidence for hats, in general, is mostly limited to caps. There are knitted examples in the Museum of London (MoL), and excavated fragments from Castle Ditch in Newcastle. From the latter, two early sixteenth-century fragments are remains of two hats of similar design to a beret; one with evidence of a brim (Walton 1981, 200, T47-50 and T51-5). Comparable knitted caps from the *Mary Rose* suggest that some may have been lined with silk (Forster *et al.* 2005, 30–4, Fig. 2.7, no. 81A0904). Two silk coifs were also found on the *Mary Rose*, one belonging to the barber-surgeon (*ibid.*, 26). The straight caps mentioned in the north-east documents were probably similar to a hat (*c.* 1580–1600) in the MoL which is formed of a circle of black, patterned velvet pleated over a hard foundation (Arnold 1985, Fig. 235).[8]

Other male headwear included more privately worn paraphernalia – nightcaps. These caps, such as the late sixteenth- to early seventeenth-century silk and spangled decorated linen example in the MMA (accession no. 26.29), together with nightgowns would have been worn around the house in private and were new to society in the 1530s. John Wilkinson had a satin nightcap for sale for ij^s in his Great Shop in 1571;[9] Richard Seymour, thought to have been a domestic in Auckland Castle, gifted his nightgown to his sister in 1565;[10] Bertram Anderson, merchant of Newcastle, also had an old nightgown among his possessions in 1570 valued at xx^s;[11] and in the same year another merchant John Havelocke bequeathed his nightgown.[12] In the Verney Collection there is an extant nightgown thought to have belonged to Sir Frances Verney in the 1610s. It is made of purple silk damask, lined with slate blue silk shag and trimmed with gold and silver braid; matching pantofles and a nightcap have also survived (National Trust 1446623, Claydon House Collection). Under the nightgowns, linen night shirts would have been worn, an example with decorative embroidery thought to date from the 1580s is in the MoL collection (accession no 28.84). Hayward (2009, 337) has suggested that the nightgown would have acted as a reinforcement of status among family and friends during Henry VIII's reign. We can see from the documentary evidence that by the 1560s and '70s nightwear was becoming more usual among the wealthy merchants in the north-east, rather than limited to the noble elite. An old nightgown valued at xx^s in 1570 was equal to the value of a dozen cushions;[13] six kitchen pans;[14] a gown faced with foin (tails or fur);[15] or a cow and a calf.[16] The nightgowns were treasured and valuable possessions as their inclusion in specific bequests makes clear.

More publicly worn apparel forms many of the bequests. Work clothes, every day clothes, 'best' clothes and holy day clothes are often referred to in the wills. The definitions are a useful insight into how people identified their clothing. Executors would have required a certain familiarity with the items to differentiate between 'my best gown', 'my next best', and simply 'my gown', especially if there were no other adjectives used to identify them, such as the colour or textile.

Women itemised and bequeathed their clothing by the use of the term 'best', but also the days on which they were worn, such as on holy days or work days. Widow Elizabeth Claxton of Witton Gilbert, for example, had four gowns that she bequeathed in 1569: a 'best' gown, a 'holly day' gown, a gown edged with velvet and another gown that was open upon the breast.[17] Here we see that Elizabeth differentiates between the gowns, and that her 'best' was not the same as that worn on the holy days. She also left a kirtle 'wch I do weare vpon ye hollyday'; the holy day outfit of kirtle and gown were not however bequeathed to the same person – the costume was to be divided between An Jaxson who received the kirtle, and Margaret Ruderforthe who was given the gown. The distinction between Elizabeth's 'best', holy day and other gowns and kirtles can be investigated further by incorporating evidence of fabric values from merchant inventories.

The holy day kirtle worn by Elizabeth was made of 'chamlet' [camlet], a woven fabric with no single make up as it was a term often applied to a variety of fabrics with different fibres and textures. Originally believed to be made with camel hair, it was a Middle Eastern and Cypriot produced textile, the use of which spread from the thirteenth century onwards (Jacoby 2012, 16). Some forms of it were made with Angora goathair. There is archaeological evidence for camlets found in anaerobic conditions but remains of woven cloth made with goathair can be mistakenly identified as a loosely compacted felt (Crowfoot *et al.* 2001, 77). In London evidence shows that textiles made with goathair were being used between the eleventh and seventeenth centuries (*ibid.*). By 1530 camlets were being made by Norwich worsted weavers (Kerridge 1988, 42–4). The trade of Norwich cloths was extensive, and the use of Norwich worsted in general is well represented in the north-east wills, with at least 30 articles made from it, and 13 items of camlet, including gowns, a cassock, jackets, doublets, sleeveless jackets, and lining for gowns. In the stock of the wealthy Newcastle merchant, John Wilkinson, there were 7.5 yards of black camlet worth xiiij^s, 2.5 yards of fine worsted at v^s, and 5 yards of broad worsted at xi^s viiij^d, among many other items in his Great Shop in 1571.[18] Three samples of textile from the Castle Ditch excavations are physical remains of the fine worsted available in Newcastle; they are true medium fleece types (Walton 1981, 190–1). If Wilkinson's stock of camlet and worsteds was comparable to the material Elizabeth's kirtles were made from, we can suggest that the value of her holy day camlet kirtle was less than the worsted kirtle she owned, revealing that the holy day gear was not the best in terms of monetary value.[19] It would have been perceived as improper and immoral for Elizabeth to attend church wearing clothes that were frivolously fashionable and expensive. Women's excessive apparel in general was heavily criticised by the puritan Phillip Stubbes in his *Anatomy of Abuses* (1583). A warning against such garb and vanity, and other sins, would still have been visible on church misericords dating from the fourteenth to early sixteenth centuries (Hardwick 2011), suggesting women's apparel could often be excessive and frivolous!

In contrast to the 'holy day' items 'work clothes' listed provide a window into the types of clothing worn to work. William Hawkelsey whose will dates to 1570, was a Newcastle cook, who bequeathed his trade tools and work clothes.[20] The main work clothes were his aprons; these were listed with his other tools, including a marble pestle and mortar, a printed cookery book, a ginger bread stamp, jelly 'pokes' [hippocras],[21] and knives. Four aprons were given to individuals, one of whom was his apprentice. Another of his apprentices, Robert Dalton, was to receive the rest of his working gear not specified in the will, plus a blue jacket. Blue was a colour generally associated with apprentices and servants and this gift to an apprentice was apt; Hawkesley also gave to his servant Bartheram Shotton a blue coat of livery and the printed cookery book. Another blue doublet of camlet was given by a girdler of Newcastle, Robert Blythman to one Robert Haull, most likely his apprentice, in 1548.[22] Not only do we see evidence of the distinguishing blue among apprentices and servants, but that the cook's aprons were valued belongings, as much so as his new fish knife, and jelly 'pokes'. They were gifts to aid the professional development of the apprentices; the act of giving them shows a sense of responsibility and a relationship between masters and apprentices.

Women also bequeathed their workday clothes; unfortunately there is little detail about what work they undertook, and perhaps the word 'workday' is simply used to distinguish clothing not worn on a holy day. One example where we can surmise that a woman's workday clothes were the apparel she wore to work is Jane Haule, as we know who she worked for.

The widow Jane Haule, of the South Bailey in Durham City, left many items in her will dated 1567, including workday clothes.[23] These were 'workday raiments': a hat, cap, kerchief and a rail 'worn on workdays',[24] and another black hat. Jane had been a servant to William Bennet,[25] one of the original canons of Durham and the last prior of Finchale Priory. She leased a property which before the Dissolution had been assigned to the Almoner, and afterwards to the Chapter (Archaeo-Environment Ltd 2010, 63, 66). The work she undertook would have been likely to include cleaning, mending and laundering linens, and brushing down other garments, among other day-to-day tasks. In 1558 Jane was bequeathed a workday gown from Robert Benet, the first prebendary priest of the eleventh stall in Durham Cathedral and brother of William Bennet.[26] It appears she worked for Robert as well as his brother. Robert left Jane and two other recipients (perhaps other servants) 'an ell [45in/*c.* 114cm] of the finest linnen clothe that I haue to be euerye one of them a kirchiffe'. By 1567 Jane Haule had at least six kerchiefs in her possession, the 'best' of which she gave to Anthony Haule's wife, perhaps that which had come from Robert Benet.

Jane Haule's will and inventory add to our knowledge of how clothing was stored, and that 'best' was worn much less often than the work or holy day gear. Her two best gowns, two 'tatches' [fasteners], two worsted kirtles and a scarlet petticoat totalling iij^l were all stored in the loft above her parlour – probably in the clothes press ('close pressour') that was inventoried in the same location. This compares with the rest of the clothes in her inventory that were found in her bed chamber which were her everyday (including holy day) clothes (total 2^l 8^s 8^d). These were a gown, three petticoats, two cloth kirtles, three coats (two black and a russet), two black hats (one worn on the work day), one cap, and a further two silk hats and two caps, and her 'nappere for hir bodie' (her linen undergarments). With these clothes were her pair of coral and silver beads, two velvet purses (one of which we know from her will had gold knops), two girdles with two 'demise' (demi-girdles), two pairs of silver crockes, a pair of knives, one silk ribbon, and one pearl fillet. The four chests and five coffers found in the chamber may have stored these items, among other possessions. Jane's will and inventory are comparable and contain a great deal of information about her apparel and other possessions, and her careful and considered distribution of bequests.

As referred to in Jane Haule's will and inventory, women's petticoats, neckerchiefs, kerchiefs, caps and under caps, and napery were bequeathed and listed. Being predominantly made of linens these articles of clothing do not survive well in archaeological contexts. A few late sixteenth- and seventeenth-century coifs or caps, and kerchiefs or forehead clothes worn under the caps or hats, survive in museum collections, for example, a matching cap and triangular shaped kerchief, both embroidered with silk in the blackwork style (Fig. 7.4). They both date to the last quarter of the sixteenth century and are embroidered with a floral motif, like other surviving examples. Embroidered flowers, insects and birds within a scrolling pattern were popular in the late-sixteenth and seventeenth centuries and are found on extant English linen jackets (Nunn-Weinberg 2006). The items listed in the wills and inventories may have been similarly decorated or just plain, bleached linen.

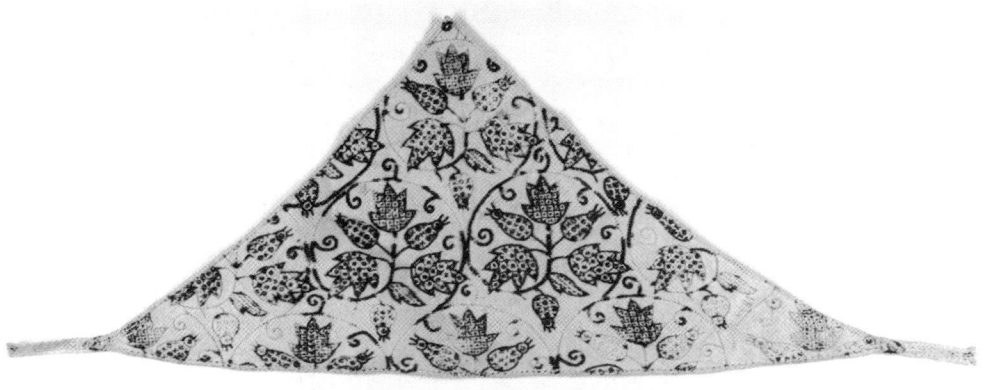

Fig. 7.4: A linen kerchief, embroidered with silk blackwork stitching. The kerchief is English and dates to c. 1575–1600. It would have been worn under a cap, such as that decorated with the same pattern also in the MMA's collection (64.101.1236). Dimensions: width 19.5in × height 7in (49.5 × 17.8cm). (©The Metropolitan Museum of Art, New York. Gift of Irwin Untermyer, 1964, accession number 64.101.1237, www.metmuseum.org).

Although clothing in these wills lack details of decoration (with the exception of religious vestments), other household furnishings are described as such: 'olde blewe cou'lng wth flouers and byrds vppon it' and a cushion with a 'pappynyay' [popinjay] on it.[27]

Clothing as gifts

By combining evidence from the wills and inventories, archaeological finds, and surviving garments in museum collections, a greater understanding of later medieval and early modern apparel can be gleaned. While the documents can give details of the physical garments that were worn in the sixteenth century, they can also provide information about the agency and significance of the gifts. The nature of gift-giving and reciprocity has provoked interest in many disciplines, and the work of Marcel Mauss, *The Gift*, is regularly cited. In medieval and early modern Europe, gifts articulated shared identities, friendship, love, esteem and support (Klein 1997; Davis 2000; O'Hara 2002; Heal 2008; Standley 2008; 2013). These are all features that can be related to the bequests of possessions in wills. Importantly the gifts acted as mnemonics reminding the recipient of these qualities and of the deceased; the clothing gifts would have physically enveloped the new owners, triggering memories of the deceased when worn.

Gifts were containers for memories and were able to create a physical link with someone no longer present. The power they possessed was associated with their previous owner and wearer in a similar fashion to clothing relics of saints. The clothing and accessories discussed above, whether kirtles, gowns, coifs or shoes embodied the benefactors for the recipients to remember. Certain items may have even taken on the physical shape of the deceased, and potentially the scent of the previous owner. Many of the senses could have been stimulated by the bequeathed clothing – sight, touch, and smell. Just as Jones and Stallybrass (2000) have highlighted that clothing could make and unmake identities in the Renaissance period, and that clothes could conjure up the dead on a stage (*ibid.*, 248), so too in a domestic context could the memory of the dead be conjured by people wearing bequeathed apparel (Standley 2013, 110–11).

Second hand or newly made goods were an addition to recipients' wardrobes, and many would have held an emotional value. The translation of gold coins into *memento mori* rings (Standley 2013, 96–8), is echoed in some of the apparel bequests. For example, pieces of clothing that were to be translated into new items, or even individual garments that were to be divided between two recipients. Symbolically the memory was transmitted within the two fragments. In functional terms, it may have also been to ensure an equal gift. Robert Blythman, the girdler from Newcastle, gave his two sisters one gown to be divided between them in 1548.[28] Both sisters could then use the material to make items for themselves, each being reminded of their brother. Other clothing bequests specified what the new items were to be; a prebendary priest, John Crawfurthe, bequeathed 'Elynor Cawsaye my worst single gown to make hir a coote off'.[29]

One accessory type imbued with significant meaning and memories were kerchiefs – they were a symbolic gift that echoed the Virgin Mary's actions. In Nicholas Love's *The Myrrour of the Blessid Life of Ihesu-Christ* (1401 translation of the thirteenth-century Franciscan text *Meditationes Vitae Christi*) Mary is reported to have wrapped the baby Christ in the kerchief from her head, and used her kerchief again to cover Christ's loins when he was on the Cross. Kerchiefs were among items that women gave to churches before the Reformation. Lowe (2010) has discussed the significance of giving textiles to parish churches and the linen kerchiefs' use as corporals on the altar. The gifts of kerchiefs to individual people would have been imbued with importance, and the agency of giving these items would have echoed the actions of the Virgin Mary in a secular context. This type of gift provides further evidence of the incorporation and transformation of meaningful and symbolic Catholic items and practices, in an essentially Protestant world (Tarlow 2003).

The symbolic aspect of giving a kerchief to a friend or relative would have embodied two of the most important aspects of Christ's life: his birth and death, and the identity and actions of the most divine female, the Virgin Mary. The physical closeness of the kerchief would have added to the personal items' social significance. Kerchiefs when worn would have covered the hair: a culturally significant part of the body (Standley 2013, 51–7). Just as posy rings, with their inner messages and reminders worn next to the skin, the kerchiefs would have held their symbolic message and reminders right next to the hair and skin of the recipient. The material itself, bleached white linen, would have also mirrored the holiness and purity of the Virgin Mary. In 1548 Janet Muschance (a widow) left the wife of Richard Chapone pieces of apparel including two velvet caps and two kerchiefs.[30] This is not an isolated case, as discussed above Jane Haule's bequests of kerchiefs are notable examples, as is the choice that Robert Benet, formerly a monk of Durham Cathedral, made in giving ells of the finest linen for kerchiefs to his three female servants. No doubt this was a conscientious choice taking into account the pious importance of the kerchief and the subtle Christian connotations in a post-Reformation context.

Gloves were another type of apparel that were regularly given as symbolic gifts in the sixteenth century, often given as wedding gifts and favours, as courtship gifts, to mourners at funerals, and as New Year's gifts. They were symbolic pieces of apparel and it is striking that they are not a popular bequest in the wills, nor do they appear in the inventories sampled. Neither does Hayward (2009, table 5.2) list them in her table of main clothing types recorded in over 1000 wills from Henry VIII's reign. The use of gloves as gifts is well documented though; they were given during courtship, and as gifts for royalty, such as the pair presented to Elizabeth I when she visited the University of Oxford in 1566 (now in the Ashmolean Museum, AN1887.1) (Rushton 1985; O'Hara 2002, 69; Ross 2008). In 1567 an envoy sent by Philip II to congratulate Duchess Giovanna de Medici on the birth of her child was given six pairs of perfumed gloves by Giovanna; and 100 pairs of gloves were given by Henry Payne to the householders in the parish of St Dunstan's on his death in 1592 (Bercusson 2009, 154; Hayward 2009, 13). In eighteenth-century New England, gifting gloves at funerals was a common and costly practice. It was deemed such an extravagant and excessive consumption, which made the state 'dangerously dependent on imported luxuries', that by the end of the century it was made illegal in Massachusetts (Bullock and McIntyre 2012, 335)!

From the 1540s onwards gloves appear more regularly in portraiture (Stallybrass and Jones 2001; Arnold 1988); their popularity in aristocratic iconography and as gifts suggest that they would appear frequently as bequests in contemporary wills. However, in the north-east sample only two men gifted gloves. One was Richard Seymour, the domestic in Auckland Castle under Bishop Pilkington, who gave Thomas Shaw a pair of red gloves, along with 'a washing ball my chest [chess] bord & chest men'.[31] And the other was Robert Conyers who left John Lanton and Thomas Clarvaux a pair of gloves each in 1431.[32] The only other gloves noted are shooting gloves, and a pair that appear in the inventory of Rauf Bouman of Durham City in 1566.[33]

Perhaps the people of the north-east did not desire to give these objects to specific recipients at their death in the second half of the sixteenth century. It cannot be that they were not owned or were seen to be culturally insignificant. They *were* used as courtship gifts and the manufacture and purchasing of gloves is evidenced by the guilds of Glovers; in Newcastle the craft company occupied part of the Blackfriars site after the Dissolution (Rushton 1985; Harbottle and Fraser 1987). Perhaps the important factor in the gifting of gloves as bequests was that they be new and unworn, or specifically made for an individual, but there were no requests to have gloves made for family members or friends in this sample of wills either. Understanding why the arena of bequests was not the place for gloves to be gifted needs further attention.

Concluding remarks

Gifting of apparel in the sample of north-east wills was a significant act, providing friends and family with personal mementos. These gifts, many with an emotional and sentimental attachment, were to perpetuate the identity of the original owner. Just as signet rings and chains embedded with families' identities were passed on as heirlooms, so too were the more ephemeral gowns, kirtles, hats and kerchiefs. The individual's memory was passed on, but also other significant memories, such as that of the Holy Family in the case of bequeathed kerchiefs.

Both women and men gave items of clothing as bequests, and not only to people of their own sex. The clothing was particularly personal, especially undergarments or apparel only worn in private, such as nightwear. Descriptions of garments as 'best' illuminate the owner's perceptions ranking and value, of clothing. With references to those clothes worn on work or holy days we can make comparisons and inferences about the actions and appearance of people. The inventories also aid our understanding of life in the home.

The documents bring to life other items of dress, for example, shoes and headgear, and the materials apparel was made from. The stock of merchants has revealed some of the articles of dress and textiles available in the north-east of England during this period. Combining contemporary excavated evidence and extant elements of costume with the documents, we can resurrect the sixteenth-century dress of a range of people from the region. While the focus here has been limited to a few garment types from a sample of wills and inventories, future studies could examine other elements of dress, household goods, retail, and the nature of bequests. Religious vestments, gloves and articles of wedding costumes are some of the possible subjects. Documentary evidence of pre-sixteenth-century date can also be combined with archaeological evidence in a similar manner.

De Vries (1993, 99) has warned that one can become lost in the wealth of information in the probate inventory, and in detailed wills, and there certainly is a wide range of information that can lead researchers into a myriad of material culture types and themes. However, the documents in Britain of sixteenth-century date, and earlier, are a resource that have so far been underused in archaeological studies and it is hoped that this chapter will help the development of a broader approach to the archaeology of dress.

Notes

1. R1835.247.
2. 1555 inventory of Sir Robert Bowes, R1835.111.
3. R1835.217.
4. R1835.274.
5. R1835.234, dated 1568.
6. R1835.150.
7. R1835.153, dated 1562.
8. For example a straight cap in R1835.159, dated 1563.
9. R1835.274.
10. R1835.165.
11. R1835.266.
12. R.1835.255.
13. Owned by Gerrerd Salveyn of Croxdale, Esquire, R1835.270.
14. Owned by Bertram, R1835.266.
15. Owned by George Smithe of Durham, R1835.260.
16. Owned by the Parson of Edmondbyers, John Foster, R1835.249.
17. R1835.248. The last gown would have revealed the clothes worn underneath, such as a kirtle and linen undershirt.
18. R1835.274.
19. Excluding the cost of tailoring. From Janet Arnold's pattern for a c. 1570–80 kirtle, c. 1.6 yards of cloth would have been required (the length of the kirtle from back neck to ground is 57.5in/146cm) (Arnold 1985, 109–11).
20. R1835.257.
21. Hippocras bags were used to filter the spiced, sugared wine used in making jellies (Brears 2010).
22. R1835.100.

23. R1835.222.
24. A rail was a garment worn about the neck made of linen or other cloth.
25. William Bennet, had been a prebendary of the fourth stall in the Cathedral. He retired to Aycliffe vicarage in 1547 (Hutchinson 1787: 184).
26. R1835.127. Robert had been a monk and bursar before the Dissolution.
27. Owned by the priest John Bynley in 1564, R1835.147.
28. R1835.100.
29. R1835.141, dated 1561.
30. R1835.95.
31. R1835.165, dated 1565.
32. R1835.56.
33. R1835.208.

Abbreviations

Ashmolean Museum = The Ashmolean Museum of Art and Archaeology, University of Oxford
MMA = The Metropolitan Museum of Art, New York
MoL = Museum of London

Bibliography

Andersson Strand, E., Frei, K. M., Gleba, M., Mannering, U., Nosch, M. L. and Skals, I. (2010) Old textiles – new possibilities. *European Journal of Archaeology* 13(2), 149–73.
Archaeo-Environment Ltd (2010) *Heritage Assessment for Proposed Developments at St John's College, The University of Durham On behalf of Derbyshire Architects and St John's College Part 1*. Barnard Castle, Archaeo-Environment Ltd.
Arkell, T., Nesta, E., and Goose, N., eds. (2000) *When Death Do Us Part: Understanding and Interpreting the Probate Records of Early Modern England*. A Local Population Studies Supplement.
Arnold, J. (1985) *Patterns of Fashion 3: The Cut and Construction of Clothes for Men and Women c. 1560–1620*. London, Macmillan.
Arnold, J., ed. (1988) *Queen Elizabeth's Wardrobe Unlock'd*. Leeds, Maney.
Bailey, G. (2007) Time perspectives, palimpsests and the archaeology of time. *Journal of Anthropological Archaeology* 26, 198–223.
Bennett, H. (1982) Textiles. In J. C. Murray (ed.) *Excavations in the Medieval Burgh of Aberdeen 1973-81*, 197–200. Edinburgh, Society of Antiquaries of Scotland (Society of Antiquaries of Scotland Monograph 2).
Bennett, H. with Muthesius, A. (1987) Textiles. In P. Holdsworth (ed.) *Excavations in the Medieval Burgh of Perth 1979–81*, 159–74. Edinburgh, Society of Antiquaries of Scotland (Society of Antiquaries of Scotland Monograph 5).
Bercusson, S. J. (2009) Gift-giving, Consumption and the Female Court in Sixteenth-Century Italy. Unpublished PhD thesis, Queen Mary College, University of London.
Biggs, C. (2007) Women, kinship, and inheritance: Northamptonshire 1543–1709. *Journal of Family History* 32(2), 107–32.
Brears, P. (2010) *Jellies and Their Moulds*. Totnes, Prospect Books.
Bullock, S. C. and McIntyre, S. (2012) The handsome tokens of a funeral: glove-giving and the large funeral in eighteenth-century New England. *The William and Mary Quarterly* 69(2), 305–46.
Burgess, C. (1987) 'By quick and by dead': wills and pious provision in late Medieval Bristol. *English Historical Review* 102, 837–58.

Burkholder, K. M. (2005) Threads bared: dress and textiles in later Medieval English wills. In R. Netherton and G. R. Owen-Crocker (eds.) *Medieval Clothing and Textiles Volume 1*, 133–54. Woodbridge, Boydell Press.

Crowfoot, E. (1975) The textiles. In C. Platt and R. Coleman-Smith, *Excavations in Medieval Southampton 1953–1969: The Finds Volume 2*, 333–40. Leicester, Leicester University Press.

Crowfoot, E. (1990) Textiles. In M. Biddle, *Object and Economy in Medieval Winchester Volume II*, 467–88. Oxford, Clarendon Press.

Crowfoot, E., Pritchard, F. and Staniland, K. (2001) *Textiles and Clothing 1150–1450 Medieval Finds from Excavations in London 4*. Woodbridge, Boydell and Brewer.

Davis, N. Z. (2000) *The Gift in Sixteenth-Century France*. Oxford, Oxford University Press.

De Vries, J. (1993) Between purchasing power and the world of goods: understanding the household economy in early modern Europe. In J. Brewer and R. Porter (eds.) *Consumption and the World of Goods*, 85–132. London, Routledge.

Deliberately Conceal Garments Project. Webpage available at: http://www.concealedgarments.org/ [accessed March 2016].

Eastop, D. (2006) Outside in: making sense of the deliberate concealment of garments within buildings. *Textile* 4(3), 238–55.

Egan, G. (2005) *Material Culture in London in an Age of Transition: Tudor and Stuart Period Finds c. 1450–c. 1700 from Excavations at Riverside Sites in Southwark*. London, Museum of London Archaeology Service (MoLAS Monograph 19).

Egan, G. and Forsyth, H. (1997) Wound wire and silver gilt: changing fashions in dress accessories c. 1400–c. 1600. In D. Gaimster and P. Stamper (eds.) *The Age of Transition: The Archaeology of English Culture*, 215–38. Oxford, Oxbow Books (Society for Medieval Archaeology Monograph 15, Oxbow Monograph 98).

Erikson, A. L. (2002) *Women and Property in Early Modern England* (2nd edition). London, Routledge.

Forster, M., Buckland, K., Gardiner, J., Green, E., Janaway, R., Klein, K. L., Mould, Q. and Richards, M. (2005) Silk hats to woolley socks: clothing remains, the textile and leather clothing assemblages. In J. Gardiner with M. J. Allen (eds.) *Before the Mast: Life and Death Aboard the Mary Rose*, 18–106. Portsmouth, Mary Rose Trust (Archaeology of the Mary Rose 4).

Gaimster, D., Hayward, M., Mitchell, D. and Parker, K. (2002) Tudor silver-gilt dress-hooks: a new class of treasure find in England. *Antiquaries Journal* 82, 157–96.

Gilchrist, R. (2009) Medieval archaeology and theory: a disciplinary leap of faith. In R. Gilchrist and A. Reynolds (eds.) *Reflections: 50 Years of Medieval Archaeology, 1957–2007*, 385–408. Leeds, Maney (Society for Medieval Archaeology Monograph 30).

Graves, C. P. and Heslop, D. H. (2013) *Newcastle upon Tyne, The Eye of the North: an Archaeological Assessment*. Oxford, Oxbow Books and English Heritage.

Grew, F. and de Neergaard, M. (2001) *Shoes and Pattens Medieval Finds from Excavations in London 2*. London, Boydell and Brewer.

Harbottle, R. B. and Fraser, R. (1987) Black Friars, Newcastle upon Tyne, after the dissolution of the monasteries. *Archaeologia Aeliana* (5th series) 15, 23–149.

Harbottle, B. and Ellison, M. with contributions by Donaldson, A. M., Robson, G. D., Rackham, J., Vaughan, J. E., and Walton, P. (1981) An excavation in the Castle ditch, Newcastle upon Tyne 1974–6. *Archaeologia Aeliana* (5th series) 9, 75–250.

Hardwick, P. (2011) *English Medieval Misericords: The Margins of Meaning*. Woodbridge, Boydell Press.

Hayward, M. (2009) *Rich Apparel: Clothing and the Law in Henry VIII's England*. Farnham, Ashgate.

Heal, F. (2008) Food gifts, the household and the politics of exchange in Early Modern England. *Past and Present* 199, 41–70.

Heley, G. (2009) *The Material Culture of the Tradesmen of Newcastle upon Tyne 1545–1642 The Durham Probate Record Evidence*. Oxford, Archaeopress (British Archaeological Report, British Series 497).

Hutchinson, W. (1787), *The History and Antiquities of the County Palatine of Durham*. London, Printed for Mr. S. Hodgson & Messrs. Robinsons.

Issa, C. (1988) Obligation and Choice: Aspects of Family and Kinship in Seventeenth Century County Durham. Unpublished PhD thesis, University of St Andrews.

Jacoby, D. (2012) Camlet manufacture, trade in Cyprus and the economy of Famagusta from the thirteenth to the late fifteenth century. In M. J. K. Walsh, P. Edbury and N. Coureas (eds.) *Medieval and Renaissance Famagusta Studies in Architecture, Art and History*, 15–42. Aldershot, Ashgate.

Jones, A. R. and Stallybrass, P. (2000) *Renaissance Clothing and the Materials of Memory*. Cambridge, University of Cambridge Press.

Kerridge, E. (1988) *Textile Manufactures in Early Modern England*. Manchester, Manchester University Press.

Klein, L. M. (1997) Your humble handmaid: Elizabethan gifts of needlework. *Renaissance Quarterly* 50(2), 459–93.

Lowe, N. A. (2010) Women's devotional bequests of textiles in the late Medieval English parish Church, c. 1350–1550. *Gender and History* 22(2), 407–29.

McKendrick, N., Brewer, J. and Plumb, J. H. (1983) *Birth of a Consumer Society: The Commercialization of Eighteenth-Century England*. London, Hutchinson.

Nunn-Weinberg, D. (2006) The matron goes to the masque: the dual identity of the English embroidered jacket. In R. Netherton and G. R. Owen-Crocker (eds.) *Medieval Clothing and Textiles Volume 2*, 151–74. Woodbridge, Boydell Press.

O'Hara, D. (2002) *Courtship and Constraint: Rethinking the Making of Marriage in Tudor England*. Manchester, Manchester University Press.

Overton, M., Whittle, J., Dean, D. and Hann, A. (2004) *Production and Consumption in English Households, 1600–1750*. London, Routledge.

Petts, D. with Gerrard, C. (2006) *Shared Visions: The North-East Regional Research Framework for the Historic Environment*. Durham, Durham County Council.

Platt, C. and Coleman-Smith, R. (1975) The leather. In C. Platt and R. Coleman-Smith, *Excavations in Medieval Southampton 1953–1969: The Finds volume 2*, 296–302. Leicester, Leicester University Press.

Raine, J., ed. (1835) *Wills and Inventories Illustrative of the History, Manners, Language, Statistics, &c., of the Northern Counties of England, from the Eleventh Century Downwards Part I*. London, J. B. Nichols and Son.

Rosenthal, M. F. (2009) Cultures of clothing in later Medieval and Early Modern Europe. *Journal of Medieval and Early Modern Studies* 39(3), 459–81.

Ross, E. (2008) 'Words, vows, gifts, tears and love's full sacrifice': an assessment of the status of Troilus and Cressida's relationship according to customary Elizabethan marriage procedure. *Shakespeare* 4(4), 397–421.

Rushton, P. (1985) The testament of gifts: marriage tokens and disputed contracts in north-east England, 1560–1630. *Folk Life* 24(1), 25–31.

Ryder, M. L. and Gabra-Sanders, T. (1992) Textiles from Fast Castle, Berwickshire, Scotland. *Textile History* 23(1), 5–22.

Spufford, M. (1976) Peasant inheritance customs and land distribution in Cambridgeshire from the sixteenth to the eighteenth centuries. In J. Goody, J. Thirsk and E. P. Thompson (eds.) *Family and Inheritance: Rural Society in Western Europe, 1200–1800*. Cambridge, Cambridge University Press.

Spufford, M. (1984) *The Great Reclothing of Rural England: Petty Chapmen and their Wares in the Seventeenth Century*. London, Bloomsbury.

Spufford, M. (2000a) Religious preambles and the scribes of villagers' wills in Cambridgeshire, 1570–1700. In T. Arkell *et al.* (eds.) *When Death Do Us Part: Understanding and Interpreting the Probate Records of Early Modern England*, 144–57. Oxford, Leopard's Head Press (Local Population Studies Supplement).

Spufford, M. (2000b) The cost of apparel in seventeenth-century England, and the accuracy of Gregory King. *The Economic History Review* 53(4), 677–705.

Stallybrass, P. and Jones, A. R. (2001) Fetishizing the glove in Renaissance Europe' *Critical Inquiry* 28(1), 114–32.

Standley, E. (2008) Ladies hunting: a Late Medieval decorated mirror case from Shapwick, Somerset. *Antiquaries Journal* 88, 198–206.

Standley, E. R. (2013) *Trinkets and Charms: The Use, Meaning and Significance of Dress Accessories 1300–1700*. Oxford, Oxford University School of Archaeology (Oxford University of Oxford School of Archaeology Monograph 78).

Swann, J. (1996) Shoes concealed in buildings. *Costume* 30(1), 56–69.

Tankard, D. (2012) 'A pair of grass-green woollen stockings': the clothing of the rural poor in seventeenth-century Sussex. *Textile History* 43(1), 5–22.

Tarlow, S. (2003) Reformation and transformation: what happened to Catholic things in a Protestant world. In D. Gaimster and R. Gilchrist (eds.) *The Archaeology of Reformation 1480-1580*, 108–21. Leeds, Maney (Society for Post-Medieval Archaeology Monograph 1).

Vaughan, J. E. (1981) The leather. In B. Harbottle *et al.* An excavation in the Castle ditch, Newcastle upon Tyne 1974–6. *Archaeologia Aeliana* (5th series) 9, 184–90.

Walton, P. (1981) The textiles. In B. Harbottle *et al.* An excavation in the Castle ditch, Newcastle upon Tyne 1974–6. *Archaeologia Aeliana* (5th series) 9, 190–228.

Walton Rogers, P. (1997) *Textile Production at 16-22 Coppergate: The Small Finds*. York, Council for British Archaeology (Archaeology of York 17).

Walton Rogers, P. (2011) Textiles. In R. Brown and A. Hardy *Trade and Prosperity War and Poverty: An archaeological and historical investigation into Southampton's French Quarter*. Oxford, Oxford Archaeology Monograph 15.

Weatherill, L. (1988) *Consumer Behaviour and Material Culture, 1660-1760*. London, Routledge.

Weatherill, L. (1993) The meaning of consumer behaviour in late seventeenth- and early eighteenth-century England. In J. Brewer and R. Porter (eds.), *Consumption and the World of Goods*, 206–27. London, Routledge.

Chapter 8

Redressing the balance: dress accessories of the non-elites in Early Modern England

Natasha Awais-Dean

On 10 July 1569, as Queen Elizabeth I (r. 1558–1603) journeyed through Eltham, she lost 'on[e] aglette of gold with a smale Rubie in it' (Arnold 1980, n. 89). This record is just one of many noting the hundreds of small jewels that fell off the clothing of the queen over the course of her progresses of the realm between 1561 and 1585. The manuscript in which these records appear (Day Book 1561–85) details the items that left the Wardrobe of the Robes, which was a small subdivision of the Great Wardrobe. In addition to itemising those jewels that were lost from the queen's person, the day book also notes material that was passed to certain ladies-in-waiting to produce accessories for Elizabeth, material and old garments given to tailors, and gifts of clothing (Arnold 1980, 9). While this information certainly enhances our understanding of processes, such as the circulation of material goods within the royal household and the networks that facilitated these movements, the entries that are most telling for the purposes of this chapter, are those small items of jewellery that became detached from Elizabeth's clothing. These accounts provide evidence of the types of objects that embellished a royal body or, more specifically, royal clothing. But, more than this, the evidence highlights the relative ease with which these jewelled dress accessories became detached from the fabrics to which they were fastened. This, in turn, explains the frequent finds of Early Modern dress accessories in archaeological and non-stratified contexts, the latter including those reported as Treasure or recorded through the Portable Antiquities Scheme (PAS). These finds provide significant evidence for the consumption of dress accessories amongst those of a lower social standing. This chapter redresses the balance, often skewed by documentary and visual sources that favour the elite, by moving away from considering Renaissance dress accessories merely as a courtly concern and instead considers the significance of less intrinsically valuable ornaments to their owners of more modest means.

All manner of ornaments could decorate the clothing of men and women in the Early Modern period. A seventeenth-century dictionary (Howell 1660) makes reference to a number of items that can be considered as embellishments to male dress. The entries reveal which types of objects were suitable for and were worn by men in the seventeenth century. Many of these relate to clothing but jewellery, dress embellishments, and associated verbs feature too, including the following: buttons, to button up, to unbutton, button loops, points, the tags of the points, to truss ones points, to untruss, a gold hat-band, and embroidered with jewels.

Many dress accessories were functional in nature, since this was a period when clothing was made of detachable parts, such as sleeves. These parts were held together by buttons, pins, points, ribbons, and hooks and eyes (Jones and Stallybrass 2000, 24). A clasp, reported as Treasure (2007 T613), undoubtedly had a functional use – to hold together parts of clothing, such as the opening of a cloak – but its decorative features indicate that it was made to imitate more costly examples. This silver-gilt fastening is decorated on the obverse with four roundels, three of which have the remains of a green substance, which is possibly enamel or a paste composition, to allude to more precious materials. Ornaments that had a functional use can be termed collectively as 'dress fastenings', since they served some use in holding together clothing. The pairs of tags or laces that we see holding together the slashing of Edward VI's (r. 1547–1553) richly embroidered red cloak in the portrait painted shortly after his accession in 1547 (National Portrait Gallery, NPG 5511) are items to be included in this category of fastenings. We must consider that within this period, the cost for the fashioning of an item of jewellery with decorative motifs and the like would have inflated the cost of the basic item. So any ornamentation or addition of materials superfluous to the function of the dress fastening added unnecessary cost for the consumer. But as the clasp above shows (along with other surviving objects and numerous visual sources), a seemingly ordinary and practical object could be, and certainly was, embellished.

Some accessories, however, were merely decorative and appear to have had no practical use. The gold triangular-shaped ornaments, each set possibly with a pearl, that adorn the cloak of the courtier Sir Christopher Hatton (c. 1540–1591) (National Portrait Gallery, NPG 2162), providing decoration to the otherwise plain, black fabric, are a case in point. In the above-cited National Portrait Gallery depiction of Edward, the young king can be seen with a number of aglets in his cap. Aglets were purely decorative, were worn in pairs to embellish hats and doublets, and were usually of cylindrical form, such as the relatively recent find of a gold aglet in Greenwich (Fig. 8.1).

The term 'dress accessories', then, encompasses a far wider range of objects than 'dress fastenings' but it is perhaps still limiting, for it positions these objects only in relation to clothing and textiles. Discounting any base-metal examples, there is sufficient evidence within the various records of Wardens' accounts and Court minutes from the Goldsmiths' Company throughout the sixteenth century to suggest that objects such as aglets, buttons, hooks, and clasps were the products of a goldsmith's output. Amongst the records of freedoms and apprentices are those fines imposed following the submission (or seizure) of sub-standard goods to the Company. For example, on Monday 26 May 1567 Thomas Pope was fined 2s for producing a 'claspe of a cloke' that was 44 penny weights below standard (Wardens' Accounts and Court Minutes, f.354). The Wardens also monitored the sale of these small-scale goods at the various fairs that took place all over England. In 1569 at the fairs of Bury in Lancashire, Harleston in Norfolk, and Woodbridge in Suffolk a variety of substandard wares were being sold by goldsmiths, which included 'claspes without hookes', 'claspes for clokes', 'pynnes', 'paires of gylte hookes', and 'paires of eyes and claspes' (Wardens' Accounts and Court Minutes, f.424). The recurrence of small-scale dress accessories seized at the fairs suggests that these were the places from which many ordinary people purchased these seemingly ubiquitous goods of gold and silver.

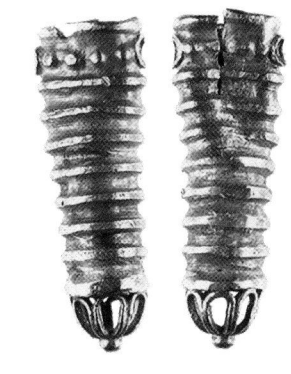

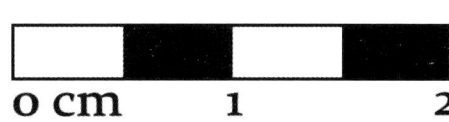

Fig. 8.1: Two views of a gold aglet with ridge and pellet decoration, found in Greenwich, Greater London; England; first half of sixteenth century, Treasure ID: 2011 T44 (PAS finds reproduced under Creative Commons Share-Alike Agreement).

To cater for an even broader range of the population wishing to adorn their items of clothing, base-metal dress accessories were available and many of these have been unearthed as archaeological finds or reported through the PAS (Table 8.1). As an example, we can see from the Portable Antiquities Scheme data presented in Table 8.1 that a simple search of certain dress accessories from the post-medieval period shows that a significant number of copper-alloy pieces have been discovered, particularly in comparison to examples declared as Treasure. These inexpensive and fairly ubiquitous items may have been available from pedlars, chapmen, and itinerant sellers, who not only operated outside of the guild system but were also mobile and ephemeral. As such, it is difficult to assess effectively the role they played within the Early Modern period. John Heywood's (1497–c. 1578) mid-sixteenth-century play offers some indication of the varied wares of a pedlar. When asked by the Apothecary about the goods he has in tow, the Pedlar enumerates some of the items that he has to sell, including dress accessories:

> 'Gloues, pynnes, combes, glasses unspottyd
> Pomanders, hooks, and lasses knotted
> Broches, rynges, and all maner bedes
> Lace rounde and flat for womens hedes
> Nedyls, threde thymbell, shers, and all suche knackes
> Where louers be no suche thynges lackes
> Sypers swathbondes rybandes and sleue laces
> Gyrdyls, knyues, purses, and pyncases' (Heywood 1545)

Table 8.1: Comparison of select categories of dress accessories from the post-medieval period between those made of copper-alloy and those declared as Treasure

Type	Copper-alloy	Treasure find
Button	2486	148
Button & loop fastener	3	0
Dress fastener (dress)	377	86
Dress fastener (unknown)	159	21
Dress hook	907	153
Dress pin	5	25
Dress stud	1	0
Lace tag	62	12
Hooked tag	1671	84

Data taken from the Portable Antiquities Scheme database on 24 August 2015.

The 'buttons of golde with diamondes', 'Agletes of gold' enamelled in all manner of colours, 'buttons of gold enameled white and blue', and 'diamond-set gold clasps' (Arnold 1980, nn. 45, 52, 53, 64, 71, 126, 248) as worn by Elizabeth and elite Renaissance citizens offer a somewhat distorted view of the types of dress accessories in circulation by focusing on elite consumption. If we shift our attention to the silver and silver-gilt ornaments typically unearthed as Treasure finds or even to the base-metal examples recorded archaeologically (Egan 2005, 39–52; Read 2005; Read 2008), it becomes clear that these objects were worn by men and women from a range of social backgrounds. In fact, searches on the PAS online database for controlled terms such as 'dress fastener', 'dress hook' or 'button' give an indication of just how commonplace such items were amongst ordinary citizens in the Early Modern period.[1] Through these archaeological records, it is possible to demonstrate that the glittering, decorative jewels worn on clothing were adopted by a broader section of the population than is perhaps suggested by Elizabeth's day book accounts, portraiture, and inventories of wealthy individuals. While there is sufficient evidence to show that these small-scale ornaments were worn by both sexes, this chapter aims specifically to understand what these objects meant to their often overlooked male owners and focuses on two objects types: the hat ornament and the button.

Hat ornaments

A 'brouche of golde' listed in the 1547 inventory of Henry VIII (r. 1509–1547) is described as being 'enameled sett with a Rock Rubie and a table diamounte with three men and a woman with a Scripture over the Rubie'. This object was worn as a hat ornament and the 'Cappe of blacke vellat', with which it is associated, was additionally 'garneshed with lxxij Buttons of golde in every Button three peerles one <perle> lacking (Starkey 1998, n. 3263). In the day book from the Wardrobe of the Robes an entry on 5 May 1574 records a gift from Elizabeth I to Thomas Sidney (1569–1595), the third son of Sir Henry Sidney (1529–1586), of 'One Cappe of blak taphata having a bande of goldesmythes worke conteyning xxv Hartes and Roses enameled and with thre litle pearles pendaunte to every harte' (Arnold 1980, n. 171). These two records reveal the types of jewels that could decorate male headgear within this period: large hat ornaments, both emblematic and not; 'buttons', which in this context are most likely to be cap-hooks; and hat bands, which seem to have been worn from the second half of the sixteenth century.

The larger, brooch-like hat ornament of the type described in Henry's inventory above was a particular object type that was popular in the sixteenth century across Europe. The noted sixteenth-century Florentine goldsmith and sculptor Benvenuto Cellini (1500–1575) observed this fashion in his autobiography: 'At this time you would use some small medals of gold, upon which each man or gentleman liked to have engraved his whim or device; and they would wear these on their hats (Cellini 1973, book 1, xxxi).[2] The ornaments described here are clearly of the emblematic type but these jewels could also be ornamented with only decorative motifs that bore no iconographical meaning. Contemporary portraiture shows both the emblematic style and purely decorative pieces affixed to the caps of elite or wealthy Renaissance men (for example, see Sir Christopher Hatton in National Portrait Gallery, NPG 2162). The hats and caps worn by men in this period were suited for the placing of such jewels. Since women were more accustomed to wearing hoods, the top of their bodies were ornamented in different ways, with pearls very often lining the edges. This can be seen on Mary Nevill, Lady Dacre (1524–c. 1576) in the double portrait by Hans Ewouts (fl.1540–1574, National Portrait Gallery, NPG 6855). As such, the use of hat ornaments as described here can be considered as a distinctly male aesthetic.

Despite their frequent depictions in contemporary images the placing of these large, brooch-like ornaments on the hat had a relatively brief history, falling out of favour by the later years of the sixteenth century. The decline in popularity of this jewel can be attributed mostly to two factors: changing fashions in headgear, favouring a taller, stiffer brimmed hat unsuitable for the placing of these ornaments; and changing aesthetics in jewellery design, moving away from the art of the goldsmith and enameller towards a preference for an abundance of gemstones, using the gold merely as a setting.

The adoption of this fashion has been attributed to the entry of the French king Charles VIII (1470–1498) and his men into Naples on 22 February 1495, from where it spread north through the Italian peninsula and into the European courts (Hackenbroch 1996, 90). This view is supported by the sixteenth-century Italian author Paolo Giovio (1483–1552), who comments on the origins of the trend for adorning the hat with jewels:

But in our times, after the arrival of King Charles VIII and Louis XII into Italy, everyone who was accustomed to following the military, in imitation of the

French captains, looked to adorn himself with fine and ostentatious emblems (Giovio 1559, A4v).[3]

While the badge of gold worn by Charles VIII was a military badge and its purpose was to allow the king to clearly distinguish himself from his army, the aesthetic was so admired that these military badges were adapted to reflect humanist thought and Renaissance ideas of self-fashioning. These Renaissance hat ornaments marked a clear shift from a military context, as they entered the secular world and became adopted by men as personal jewels.

The *Kleinodienbuch der Herzogin Anna von Bayern*, made by the court painter Hans Mielich (1516–1573) between 1552 and 1556, is a pictorial inventory that records the jewels owned by Albrecht V (1528–1579), duke of Bavaria and his wife Anna (1528–1590). Amongst the 108 illuminations, 71 jewelled possessions are depicted. Three of these are hat jewels and they are gold, enamelled, and set with faceted diamonds. They offer parallels with extant survivals and so propagate further the perception that Renaissance hat ornaments were part of an elite aesthetic, a view that is strengthened by many documentary and visual sources, such as we have seen above. The material evidence, however, offers us a much broader perspective and allows us to consider the wearing of these hat ornaments lower down the social scale. A number of Limoges enamelled roundels or plaques can be identified as jewels worn in the hat. To substantiate this supposition, we are able to turn to a written source. The French artist and potter Bernard Palissy (1510–1589) commented on this trend in his treatises:

I am certain of having seen to give for three sols the dozen figures for *enseignes* that were worn on hats. These *enseignes* were so well worked and their enamels so well fused on the copper, that there was never any painting so pleasant (Palissy 1880, 374).[4]

Cheaper to purchase than gold jewels, objects of this type were probably worn by urban gentlemen. Yet these hat ornaments could not match the effect created by gold examples with their contrasts of high and low relief. Nevertheless, for men of more humble means, these pieces provided them with a way of accessing the latest sixteenth-century fashion at a fraction of the cost. Such men were not only restricted to the less dynamic, two-dimensional form of the enamelled roundel, for the relief decoration of the gold hat ornaments could be replicated in base metal.

Within the collections of the British Museum is a group of copper-alloy plaquettes. These were given by the collector Thomas Whitcombe Greene (1842–1932) in 1915. Amongst these bronze ornaments is a discrete group of eleven roundels that can be attributed as hat ornaments (Fig. 8.2, see Awais-Dean 2012, 170 and appendix B, 340–1), providing strong evidence of this fashion reaching a broader social spectrum than is suggested by contemporary portraiture and other visual sources.[5]

These bronze objects have certain attributes that show affinity with the high-status, gold, brooch-like hat ornaments worn by elite men (Fig. 8.3): they are circular in form and their borders are often pierced with holes to enable fastening to a cap; each object is either gilded or has traces of gilding; they are of comparable size

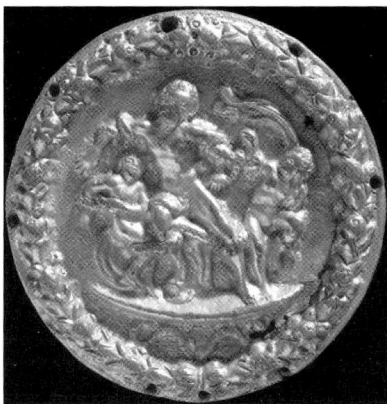
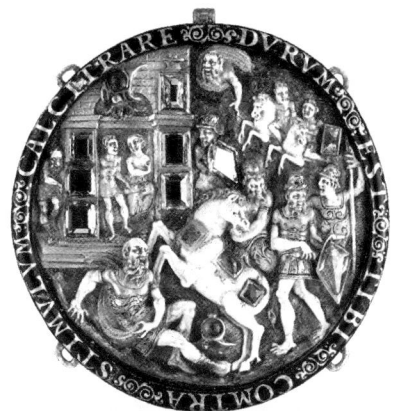

Fig. 8.2: Cast and gilded bronze hat ornament depicting Laocoon and his son overcome by a serpent, enclosed within a floral wreath border pierced with eight holes; diameter, 4.75cm; weight, 23g; Italy; sixteenth century. British Museum, 1915,1216.134 (image courtesy of the Trustees of the British Museum).

Fig. 8.3: Gold and enamelled hat ornament set with diamonds, rubies, and possibly a garnet showing the Conversion of Saul; Italy or Spain; mid-sixteenth century. British Museum, WB.171 (image courtesy of the Trustees of the British Museum).

to the precious metal examples; and they imitate stylistically the emblematic hat jewels, with the depiction of a symbolic image. Though while the precious metal examples bear imagery that can find its origins in mythology, allegory, religion, or even politics, these bronze pieces depict scenes from classical antiquity, with the exception of one showing St Matthew writing his gospel.[6] The vast majority of these gilt-bronze ornaments have been cast. This would have facilitated the production of multiple copies with relatively minimal labour costs once the mould had been made. This 'mass production' meant that they would have been available and affordable to men of a lower social standing. Once gilded and enamelled these bronze plaquettes revealed very little, if any, of the base-metal surface.

Objects such as these would have been virtually indiscernible from the gold hat jewels so popular with rulers and noblemen, when placed on a dark coloured hat at the apex of the body. For a man who could not afford ornaments of precious metal, these bronze equivalents provided a way for him to participate in contemporary fashions. These copper-alloy plaquettes, clearly intended to be ornaments for the hat, have been crucial in revealing that this particular fashion was not merely a courtly concern. The same is true of the smaller 'buttons' or cap-hooks that are referred to in Henry VIII's inventory above.

Cap-hooks were smaller in scale than the larger, brooch-like hat ornaments. Examples of gold are frequently depicted adorning the hats of English courtiers, such as Sir Nicholas Poyntz (1510–1557) (National Portrait Gallery, NPG 5583), sheriff of Gloucestershire or members of the landed gentry like Simon George of Cornwall (Städel Museum, Frankfurt, inv. no. 1065) but their ubiquitous nature amongst lower social groups was not truly appreciated until fairly recently. Since the implementation of the *Treasure Act* on 24 September 1997 there has been a significant increase in the number of reported finds of ornaments that were worn in the hat. These finds have allowed for a new understanding of this object type and have offered a different perspective about such items of jewellery than previously thought. Examples in silver, sometimes gilded, that seek to emulate more costly materials have provided material evidence that supports the non-elite wearing of such jewels.

A composite, cast parcel-gilt ornament in the form of a six-spoked Catherine-wheel is set with a multi-petalled flower-head emanating from a central hemispherical boss. Clearly intended to be decorative in nature, the effect of the contrasting colours, achieved through the partial gilding to the rim and the central boss, adds to its aesthetic qualities. The prominent central boss may have been an attempt to imitate more costly materials, such as a pearl. Based on pictorial evidence of courtly men with their gold hat ornaments, it is unlikely that an object of this type was worn in isolation: it is much more probable that this cap-hook was one of a set. Another hat ornament in the British Museum was cast in the form of a stylised flower with four petals, which are interspersed with smaller petals (British Museum, 2006,0301.1). Found in Arreton on the Isle of Wight, this piece is made of silver and has been gilded, though much of the gilding is now worn. In the centre of this cap-hook is a pyramidal form, which may be an attempt to mimic the facets of a point-cut diamond or another precious or semi-precious gemstone. It is likely that it was originally one of a set placed around the circumference of a cap. This type of ornamental cap-hook is very similar in style to the gold examples worn by Nicholas Poyntz (see NPG 5583). A final example is a circular, silver-gilt cap-hook cast entirely in one piece that has eight knops projecting from the edges and is embellished to the front with a Tudor rose (British Museum, 2009,8037.1). It is very likely that this piece was worn in a man's cap to show allegiance to the Tudor dynasty.

There has been much written about the trickle-down effect since Veblen (1899) put forward this theory, and it has certainly been applied to the Early Modern period (McKendrick *et al.* 1982) and the diffusion and consumption of fashion at this time (see, for example, Allerston 2000, 367–70). More recently, however, this view has been challenged, moving away from the idea that elite fashions were only ever replicated cheaply by the lower classes in an attempt to emulate their superiors, and towards a view that ordinary men and women could participate directly in new fashions creating their own meanings and practices far removed from the court (Hohti 2017, 165). There is no evidence as yet to suggest that the cap-hooks unearthed as Treasure or the bronze plaquettes worn as hat ornaments were produced only in imitation of fashions at court. As we have seen, the trend for the wearing of badges in the hat as ostentatious display seems to have been inspired by the military badges of the

French king Charles VIII and his army. Seen by all citizens, regardless of class, these ornaments shifted into a secular context and would have been appropriated by men from across the social spectrum.

Treasure finds, such as those discussed above, have been crucial in providing this new understanding of the use of hat jewels. Pictorial representations and many extant pieces of gold and other precious materials have propagated the belief that such items were reserved for an elite class of men. Yet, the material evidence suggests otherwise. The contemporary fashion for the wearing of hat ornaments was clearly accessed by men across the social scale.

Buttons

Buttons are an object type that has been largely neglected, despite their ubiquitous nature within visual and documentary sources. According to Jones and Stallybrass (2000, 24), in the Early Modern period there was a notable increase in the use of buttons by men and not just amongst courtiers. They cite the mid-seventeenth-century play, *The Old Law*, in which a courtier derides the fact that older men were participating in fashion: 'They love a doublet thats three houres a buttoning'.

The Museum of London has a vast collection of buttons, comprising the largest collection of medieval and Early Modern examples in the country. The majority of these buttons were discovered on the Thames foreshore by the late Tony Pilson, who donated them in 2009 along with a vast number of cufflinks. A number of materials are represented: silver, pewter, and copper-alloy, amongst others. Form, construction, and decorative features vary too. These archaeological data further our understanding of how widespread the use of buttons was within the Early Modern period. It moves us away from considering these as high-status objects of the type that were discovered within the Spanish Armada wreck, the *Girona*. Eighteen gold buttons in various states of condition – most are misshapen or flattened – were recovered from this site. Many have worn surface decoration and it has been possible to identify those that were originally part of a set and so worn together.

Further evidence of elite use is provided pictorially, such as in the extant portrait of William Herbert (1507–1570), first earl of Pembroke at Wilton House, Wiltshire, in which buttons fasten the sleeves of Pembroke's cloak and the front of his doublet; in the portrait of the courtier Henry Carey (1526–1596), first Baron Hunsdon, dated to 1591 when Carey was 66 years of age, which shows at least 20 gold filigree buttons; and in the portrait of Robert Dudley (1532–1588), earl of Leicester, which shows Leicester's doublet closed with fastenings or buttons with either a cluster of pearls or white enamelled knops placed within gold settings (Wallace Collection, P534). Amongst the drawings of jewels by Hans Holbein the Younger (1497/98–1543) from the 'Jewellery Book' (British Museum, Sloane MS 5308) are three small circular designs that were probably intended as buttons and further designs for five more ornate buttons. These drawings most likely represent jewels owned or commissioned by Henry VIII and as such are an important visual source for documenting high-status objects that are no longer extant.

Interestingly, survivals of buttons from archaeological and non-stratified contexts far outweigh any high-end examples, offering a less elite perspective of such objects. Finds recovered from the wreck of the *Mary Rose*, a favourite warship of Henry VIII that sank in the Solent in 1545, include at least 30 buttons (Gardiner and Allen 2005, 96). These would have been worn by the sailors, soldiers, and officers on board the ship. Many of these buttons comprised sets that can be associated with particular garment types. The majority of these buttons are made of wood with a silk covering but there are two examples made of leather. Seven buttons were found still affixed to three jerkins, while a single button was present on each of a shoe and an ankle boot. These finds reveal how commonplace such accessories were amongst men within the sixteenth century, constituting personal adornment that served both a functional and ornamental use.

The quantity of archaeological material has allowed for type series of buttons to be made and Read (2005) has published his findings to assist with dating and identification. For the post-medieval period, Read defines 24 types, ranging from 'cast one-piece copper-alloy buttons with integral drilled shanks', mostly cast with relief decoration, to 'die-stamped composite three-piece sheet copper-alloy buttons with separate soldered drawn copper-alloy wire shanks', mostly with engraved decoration (Read 2005, 30–97). Excavations in London, undertaken as part of the London Bridge City redevelopment from 1986 to 1999, yielded a number of base-metal buttons including copper-alloy pieces with either solid cast heads or sheet heads and lead/tin examples with solid heads and integral loops for attachment (Egan 2005, nn.178–219).

Buttons are also reported as Treasure. They represent ownership and consumption at a level higher than the archaeological material, and were possibly the possessions of relatively wealthy urban citizens outside of courtly circles. However, the number of buttons within the Treasure reports constitutes a relatively small proportion of overall post-medieval Treasure finds (Table 8.2). The table includes a separate field for cufflinks, since it seems to be significant that, in the 2009 report, there are 15 post-medieval examples reported. This is a substantial increase in previous years, when either a single instance was recorded or none at all. This could be as a result of the biases inherent within metal-detecting practices, in particular recovery, reporting, and recording (Robbins 2012, 25–7 and 36–48) or, alternatively, this could be due to better recognition. Overall, it is clear that buttons are not as frequent Treasure finds as other types of dress accessories. Apart from the 2005/2006 period when they constituted almost 23% of all post-medieval finds, on the whole gold or silver examples of this object type do not appear to be particularly common. This is somewhat startling when we consider the visual evidence. Portraits reveal that buttons were worn, when the clothing dictated it, in great numbers upon the body – never in isolation – and so we might expect to see more discovered as Treasure. The quantity of archaeological material of this object type is vast and so the relative dearth of Treasure finds does

Table 8.2: Breakdown of buttons, cufflinks, and dress accessories reported as Treasure from September 1997 to the end of 2009

Treasure Annual Report	Buttons	Cufflinks	Dress accessories	Total post-medieval finds declared to be Treasure
1997/1998	2	1	0	23
1998/1999	0	0	17	78
2000	2	0	15	65
2001	2	0	5	49
2002	1	0	13	44
2003	5	0	14	100
2004	10	0	30	116
2005/2006	31	1	73	136
2007	0	1	6	195
2008	5	1	21	207
2009	12	15	32	202

seem surprising. Nevertheless, this could simply raise more issues of biases within the dataset that begin with initial loss or discard of the material culture (Robbins 2012, 25–9).

By far the most prolific designs that appear mostly as stamped decoration on the obverse of the Treasure buttons are those that have possible associations with the marriage of Charles II (r. 1660–1685) to Catherine of Braganza (1638–1705) in 1662.[7] Data taken from the reports published from 1998 to 2009 revealed three distinct designs: two hearts (sometimes conjoined) crowned (Fig. 8.4); joined hands above two hearts, which are surmounted by a crown; and a single flaming heart pierced by two crossed arrows. Of these the crowned hearts imagery was the most common. Lewis (2013) has analysed finds bearing this 'crown and heart' motif up to 31 December 2012 and has identified three additional types to those listed above: clasped hands above two flaming hearts; two cherubs supporting a crown over a flaming heart; and a quatrefoil with four loops between which sit four hearts. These designs also appear on cufflinks. For example, two cufflinks bear a flaming heart pierced by two arrows (2006 T499 and 2008 T741), while another cufflink has the two hearts crowned motif (2007 T77). While many of the buttons with the 'crown and heart' design are silver (Lewis 2013, 2), there are examples in base metal. Two copper-alloy buttons, which were reported in 2004 and subsequently declared not Treasure, are ornamented with conjoined hearts crowned (2004 T212 and 2004 T213). These base-metal versions of a popular accessory provide strong evidence for similar fashions being enjoyed across varied social levels. So while visual evidence documents elite male use of buttons made from precious metals and materials, surviving objects from

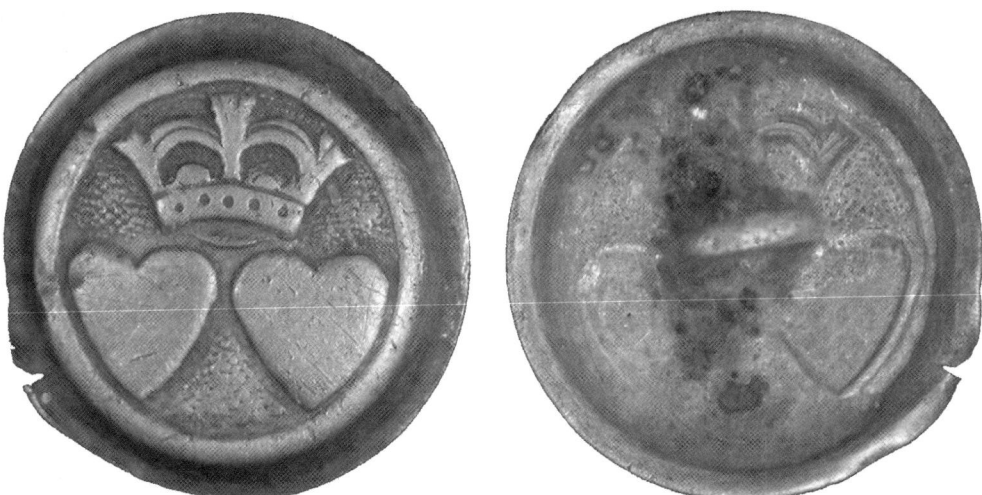

Fig. 8.4: Silver button stamped on the obverse with two hearts surmounted by a crown, found in an unknown parish, Norfolk. Diameter: 16mm; England; late seventeenth–eighteenth century [Treasure ID: 2006 T532i] (PAS finds reproduced under Creative Commons Share-Alike Agreement).

archaeological contexts give proof of usage lower down the social scale. Simpler silver and silver-gilt examples of buttons may have been worn by middle-class men or urban citizens, while the base-metal pieces were reserved for men of minimal means. That these intrinsically low-value items could still be ornamented in a way similar to the precious metal buttons demonstrates that these were still important objects within a man's possession.

Emotional values

The records of Queen Elizabeth's lost jewels show how easily dress accessories fell off clothing. These objects could also be and certainly were deliberately removed and circulated between items of clothing. References to these small-scale jewels in the wills and inventories (probate and household) of Early Modern men and women underscore their importance as personal goods. In particular, bequests of such objects suggest that to their owners, of all social standings, these goods had an emotional value that often belied their fiscal worth (see Standley this volume).

Dress accessories have been somewhat neglected by jewellery historians, since references to them are very often buried away within manuscript sources that betray no hint of their inclusion. For example, the post-mortem inventory of the parliamentarian army officer Robert Devereux (1591–1646), third earl of Essex, which begins with 'An Inventorie of the wearing apparell <w[i]th some other small things {....}>' (Devereux 1646, f.150), deals predominantly with clothing and textiles and there is no separate section listing jewels. However, there are some entries for jewelled possessions including 'A rich gold & siluer Belt Embroydred' and 'one gold & siluer hatbande' (Devereux 1646, ff.150–150v). Of particular interest is the presence of 'A <french> scarlet Cloke lined w[i]th ba{...} w[i]th siluier & gold buttons Clopes' (Devereux 1646, f.151). Likewise, in the post-mortem inventory of Henry Howard (1540–1614), Earl of Northampton, a reference to small-scale dress accessories is to be found in amongst the clothing: 'Item a white sattin dublett unlaced cutt and raced with flowers and silver buttons' (Shirley 1869, 367). Further, it is an inventory of the plate had by the courtier Sir Henry Sidney when in Ireland in September 1575 and in the possession of George Arglas that reveals that he had 'Two dozen points with silver tags' (Kingsford 1925, 276).

The household inventory of William Herbert is dated to 1561 and includes a section listing his 'Buttons and aglettes beinge on no garmentes' (Pembroke 1561, ff.73–73v). This suggests that these particular jewels were not associated with specific garments and were considered as movable objects in their own right – not merely ornamentation to an item of dress. There are also numerous records of precious metal buttons within the inventory that do appear within the context of clothing. For example, the first jerkin that is listed is described as being of 'white perfumed leather laide on thicke with a lace of black silke, golde and silver, lyned with blacke taffata with xxv knott buttons of golde, white and black enameled' (Pembroke 1561, f.48r). Another black satin jerkin is 'sett with ii dosen ii golde buttons snaile fashion, white enameled' (Pembroke 1561, f.48r). These buttons in the form of a snail also feature on a black satin doublet (Pembroke 1561, f.51r).

In fact, Pembroke was in possession of a vast array of buttons which were presumably circulated between his clothing. The buttons are listed by type and this indicates that they were worn in sets, with Herbert owning at least 11:

> 'Vlviii buttons enameled blewe and redde w[i]th iii perles on every button.
> Item xxxvi buttons of golde black enameled
> Item vi dosen buttons, white and blewe enameled fasshioned like the sonne.
> Item iii dosen and x buttons enameled white and black w[i]th iiii corners.
> Item xlii buttons w[i]th iii perles on every button beinge black enameled.
> Item lxviii buttons of golde
> Item xxii buttons lesser like vnto the same.
> Item iii dosen iiii buttons enameled white called Pannses made by Denham.
> Item v buttons white and black enameled
> Item iiii buttons made like snailles enameled white
> Buttons
> Item ii dosen viii greate buttons bosselike w[i]th a faire perle on the toppe of every button enameled white black and blewe' (Pembroke 1561, ff.73–73v)

The fact that the majority of Pembroke's jerkins and doublets had buttons attached to them suggests that those buttons not associated with clothing must have been particularly special items. They were presumably affixed to his dress when the occasion demanded it. This practice of keeping buttons separate from clothing seems to have been adopted by non-elite men as well. The sailor Edward Barnes, whose inventory is dated 14 March 1590, owned twenty-four silver buttons (Reed 1981, 30–1). The manner of recording these objects suggests that Barnes in fact owned two distinct sets, each comprised of 12 buttons. It is likely that Barnes wore these silver buttons on special occasions, removing them from his clothing when he was at sea.

Inventories of ordinary Early Modern citizens, unsurprisingly, suggest that very few individuals owned items of jewellery or dress accessories. Of those who did possess such goods, these items comprise a small percentage of their entire inventoried estate. It is important to note, however, that inventories can never provide information about objects that were not present when the appraisers valued the goods of an individual, and so any bequeathed goods alienated prior to an inventory being taken remain unknown. Given the highly personal nature of these objects, it is not beyond possibility that men would choose to pass on whatever little jewellery (including dress accessories) they owned to family and friends, removing them from these probate records. Inventories for the male inhabitants of the town of Ipswich that date from 1583 to 1631 (Reed 1981) provide an indication of ownership beyond a courtly context. Analysis of the 59 published inventories suggests that rings and small dress accessories were the most common items owned by these men and this is a reflection of what occurs at higher levels of society.

As further indication of ownership trends amongst the lower classes it is possible to turn to testamentary evidence. More than serving as a mere indicator of the types of goods a person owned, as manifest in inventories, bequests highlight the significance that bequeathed objects may have had for their owners. Further, these documents provide crucial insight into the relationships forged throughout an individual's lifetime. The memory of the deceased that was evoked in the bequeathing of material artefacts was intensified through the bequest of jewels, since the highly personal nature of these small-scale objects and the proximity to the body only served to increase the status of these gifts. So while inventories can provide documentary evidence of actual ownership of these smaller jewels (when present), showing that they were deemed worthy enough of recording, wills provide more effective evidence of the range of values that dress accessories had for their owners.

The will of Robert Steyll, chaplain of St Mary Woolchurch in London, dated to 1 August 1510 gives insight into the limited possessions of a religious figure (Darlington 1967, n.12). There are a number of monetary bequests, ranging from four pence left to Ralph Bransby to 3l 6s 8d which is given to James Fynard, a citizen and goldsmith of London and one of Steyll's executors. Additionally Fynard receives Steyll's 'best cap'. These are in addition to a further 20s given to Fynard in his capacity as executor. The second executor, Simon Fowlar, also receives 20s for his role but he too is remembered in the will. He receives from Steyll his 'best cloak and a tippet and two clasps of silver and a breviary'. It is likely that these two clasps were worn exclusively with this best cloak and tippet. Excepting the monetary gifts the majority of bequests are of clothing, save also for Steyll's bed, its furnishings, and chamber hangings, which he leaves to a kinsman by the name of Thomas. It is clear then that Steyll is leaving to his family and friends all that was dear to him. The two silver clasps that Fowlar receives are amongst the few items listed that are not clothing. A fellow chaplain, John Upton, is fortunate to receive the only other jewel – 'a silver clasp with a crucifix'. The only other object made of precious metal is a silver spoon and this is left to Richard Atkynson, along with a primer of parchment. That Steyll saw fit to bequeath the three silver clasps he owned, rather than having them sold to pay for the provisions in his will, suggests that they were personal to him and that he wished for their reuse by individuals close to him.

In contrast, the parson of Nevendon in Essex, Thomas Awsten, was more concerned over his mother's wellbeing. He left the vast majority of his estate to his brother Rychard Awstyn in order to provide for their mother (Darlington 1967, n. 65). However, Thomas does make two named bequests in his will of 10 July 1518. These are both of a 'tache of sylver and gilt'. A 'tache' is an obsolete and generic term used to describe something that fastens two parts together, so this would include objects such as clasps, buckles, and hooks and eyes. The first is left to provide for his parish church 'for to make a howke for the pyx over the high alter ther'. The second is given to Thomas Tendryng, along with a girdle of black silk. Again, while one of these taches is considered only for its monetary worth, Awsten still sees fit to give one to his acquaintances rather than take advantage of its fiscal value for his mother's care.

Another man, Thomas Bellamy, in his will dated to 11 August 1518 leaves his witness Robert Hill his best gown, a gelded colt, and a tippet of sarsenet 'with my tache of silver' (Darlingon 1967, n. 68). Bellamy's occupation is not stated but he bequeaths a number of animals and quantities of hay, which suggests that he was a farmer. The remainder of his named bequests include clothing, bedding, and vessels of pewter and these goods suggest that his means were relatively limited. So, along with a single silver spoon bequeathed to his brother Roger Belamy the silver tache constituted his only precious metal possessions and indeed his only item of jewellery.

The will of the widow Anie Diryckson, dated to 17 September 1541, provides evidence of goods that were presumably the possession of her late husband in the form of a bequest to a certain Garret Kirikell of 'his unculles beste gowne, beste jacket of worsted, blacke cloke and 40s.' (Darlington 1976, n. 144). So it is unclear whether the bequest of a 'peare of sylver hokes' to her cousin Neskyn were items of her personal use or originally belonged to her husband. Nevertheless, this record still shows that these very small items, used to hold clothing together, were valuable possessions to the men and women who owned them. Through the documentary records of less wealthy Early Modern men and women it is clear that small proportions of them did own dress accessories but the numbers they owned were small. Nonetheless they were highly significant to the men and women who owned and used them.

Bequests of small dress accessories (and other jewels) allow us to understand better the emotional worth of these objects. Since they were highly personal possessions they provided a potent and tangible reminder of the deceased. The movement of these goods to family and friends signalled and reinforced the bonds of kinship forged over a lifetime. It is not only the bequeathed article that holds a value but also the recipient of the gift. And so in 1527 the Lincolnshire mercer John Leek leaves a number of items, including his wife's wedding ring, to Alice Arley (Awais-Dean 2012, 274). The ring served as a tangible reminder of Leek, his wife, and their union. This symbolically-charged bequest suggests that Alice Arley was a highly valued kinswoman.

In addition to creating strong ties of remembrance between the testator and the recipient, some jewelled goods were bequeathed as heirloom pieces with the intention of creating a powerful sense of family heritage. In this way, the originator of the bequest becomes memorialised in a gift. This gift then becomes the embodiment of the testator's posterity through his male descendants. This practice is eloquently described by William Shakespeare in his play *All's Well That Ends Well*. Diana requests Bertram's ancestral ring, as a token of his affection but he refuses:

> 'I'll lend it thee, my dear; but have no power
> To give it from me.
> [...]
> It is an honour 'longing to our house,
> Bequeathed down from many ancestors
> Which were the greatest obloquy i'the world
> In me to lose.'

Bertram is unable to alienate himself from this ring, for it symbolises simultaneously patrilineage, family memory, and his own individual identity.[8] In this instance, the ring has become something far greater than simply a bequest from one individual to another. It now has a resonance stronger than any man who might come to possess it. This literary offering merely echoes contemporary practice and Shakespeare would have been mindful of this. There do not appear to be any sources that document this occurring at the level of ordinary citizens but there is evidence of the creation of heirloom pieces taking place amongst the elite, with the will of the statesman Sir Thomas Sackville (c. 1536–1608) being just one such example (see Awais-Dean 2012, 284-7). While we are unlikely to find a man of more modest means being explicit in forming heirloom pieces through any jewelled goods he might bequeath, it would not be unreasonable to suppose that some bequests of jewellery (including dress accessories, such as buttons) may have been deemed worthy enough to be retained over generations.

Conclusion

Small-scale dress accessories made of precious and base metals constituted items of jewellery within the Early Modern period. They adorned male and female dress, providing both ornamental and functional use but this chapter has focused specifically on the male body. Archaeological finds in stratified and non-stratified contexts, including items reported as Treasure and those recorded within the PAS database, have allowed for a new understanding of dress accessories. Represented pictorially within the painting of elite Tudor men, these objects have traditionally been considered as being for the exclusive reserve of courtiers and noblemen. Yet, the often-gilded silver jewels worn as hat ornaments and so similar in style and form to the gold and gem-set jewels worn by the elite suggest otherwise. Buttons clearly intended for use by individuals of more modest means, most with engraved or stamped decoration, provide evidence that function was not the only concern when purchasing such goods. The presence of these dress accessories within inventories and wills highlights their relative importance to Early Modern citizens across all social scales. By focusing on consumption of the non-elites, only made possible through the incorporation of archaeological data, it is clear that Renaissance dress accessories were valued by their male owners for more than their fiscal worth. The values that a man assigned to his jewels were no less significant whether he were a nobleman or a man of more modest means.

Notes

1. A search carried out on the Portable Antiquities Scheme database on 24 August 2015 yields the following results for post-medieval material: 'button', 3500; 'dress fastener (dress)', 488; 'dress fastener (unknown)', 185; and 'dress hook', 1114. These figures include all base-metal and Treasure items within these categories.
2. 'Se usava in questo tempo alcune medagliette d'oro, che ogni signore e gentiluomo li piaceva fare scolpire in esse un suo capriccio o impresa; e le portavano nella berretta' – English translation is author's own.
3. 'Ma à questi nostri te[m]pi dopò la venuta del Rè Carlo Ottauo e di Lodouico XII in Italia, ogn'vn, che seguitaua la militia, imitando i Capitani Francesi, cercò di adornarsi di belle e pompose Imprese' – English translation is author's own.
4. 'Je m'assure avoir vu donner pur trois sols la douzaine des figures d'enseignes que l'en portoit aux bonnets, lasquelles enseignes estoyent si bieng labourées et leurs esmaux si bien parfondus sur le cuivre, qu'il n'y avoit nulle peinture si plaisante' – English translation is author's own with assistance from Corinne Thepaut-Cabasset, formerly of the Victoria and Albert Museum.
5. British Museum registration numbers: 1915,1216.125; 1915,1216.128; 1915,1216.130–136; 1915,1216.226; and 1915,1216.298.
6. British Museum 1915,1216.226.
7. This connection seems to have first been put forward by Ivor Noël Hume in *A Guide to Artifacts of Colonial America* (Philadelphia, University of Pennsylvania Press, 1969), p. 89, fig. 22. Gaimster and Thornton put forward this theory with the first recorded Treasure example of this type found in Rochester, Kent in 2001 (British Museum 2002,0711.1). Lewis (2013) acknowledges that the motif did appear prior to the 1662 marriage but seems to have had religious connections. This association is not confirmed however and, in the absence of any known documentary sources, this is mere hypothesis. Brian Read also acknowledges that this link between the motif and the royal marriage is only supposition (personal correspondence (27/08/2015).
8. For a full discussion of this exchange, see Awais-Dean 2012, 277–9.

Bibliography

Allerston, P. (2000) Clothing and Early Modern Venetian Society. *Continuity and Change* 15(3), 367–90.

Arnold, J., ed. (1980) *'Lost from Her Majesty's Back': Items of Clothing and Jewels Lost or Given Away by Queen Elizabeth I between 1561 and 1585, Entered in One of the Day Books Kept for the Records of the Wardrobe of Robes*. London, Costume Society.

Awais-Dean, N. (2012) Bejewelled: the Male Body and Adornment in Early Modern England. Unpublished PhD thesis, Queen Mary, University of London.

Cellini, B. (1973) *La Vita* (edited by Guido Davico Bonino). Turin, Nuova Universale Einaudi.

Darlington, I., ed. (1967) *London Consistory Court Wills 1492-1547*. London, London Record Society.

'Day book of Queen Elizabeth's wardrobe of robes', 1561–1585 (Duchess of Norfolk's Deeds), National Archives, London C 115/91 nos 6697.

Devereux (1646) 'Household Inventory of Robert Devereux, 3rd Earl of Essex (1596–1646)'. British Library, Additional MS 46189, ff.150–65.

Egan, G. (2005) *Material Culture in London in an Age of Transition, Tudor and Stuart Period Finds c. 1450-c. 1700*. London, Museum of London Archaeological Service.

Gaimster, D., Hayward, M., Mitchell, D. and Parker, K. (2002) Tudor silver-gilt dress-hooks: a new class of treasure find in England. *Antiquaries Journal* 82, 157–96.

Gardiner, J. and Allen, M. J. eds. (2005) *Before the Mast: Life and Death Aboard the Mary Rose*. Portsmouth, Mary Rose Trust (Archaeology of the Mary Rose 4).

Giovio, P. (1559) *Dell'Imprese Militari Et Amorose Di Monsignor Giovio Vescouo Di Nocera; Con Un Ragionamento Di Messer Lodouico Domenichi, Nel Medesimo Soggetto*. Lyon, Guglielmo Roviglio.

Hackenbroch, Y. (1996) *Enseignes: Renaissance Hat Jewels*. Florence, Studio per edizioni scelte.

Heywood, J. (1545, reproduced in facsimile 1908) *The Play Called the Four PP* (edited by John S. Farmer). London, Tudor Facsimile Texts.

Hohti, P. (2017) Dress, dissemination and innovation: artisan fashions in sixteenth- and early seventeenth-century Italy. In E. Welch (ed.) *Fashioning the Early Modern: Dress, Textiles and Innovation in Europe, 1500-1800*, 143–165. Oxford, Pasold Research Fund/Oxford University Press.

Howell, J. (1660) *Lexicon Tetraglotton, an English-French-Italian-Spanish Dictionary: Whereunto Is Adjoined a Large Nomenclature of the Proper Terms (in All the Four) Belonging to Several Arts and Sciences, to Recreations, to Professions Both Liberal and Mechanik, &C. Divided into Fiftie Two Sections; with Another Volume of the Choicest Proverbs*. London, J. G. for Cornelius Bee.

Jones, A. R. and Stallybrass, P. (2000) *Renaissance Clothing and the Materials of Memory*. Cambridge, Cambridge University Press.

Kingsford, C. L., ed. (1925) *Report on the Manuscripts of Lord De L'Isle & Dudley Preserved at Penshurst Place* (6 volumes). London, HMSO.

Lewis, M. (2013) *'Crown and Heart' Buttons and Cufflinks*. London, The Finds Research Group AD 700–1700 (Datasheet 46).

McKendrick, N., Brewer. J. and Plumb, J. H. (1982) *The Birth of a Consumer Society: The Commercialization of Eighteenth-Century England*. London, Europa Publications.

Palissy, B. (1880) *Les Oeuvres*. Paris, Charavay Frères.

Pembroke (1561) 'Inventory of Gold and Silver Plate, Jewells and Apparrell Etc. Of William, Earl of Pembroke', 12 December 1561, National Art Library, MSL/1982/30.

Read, B. (2005). *Metal Buttons, c. 900 BC-c. AD 1700*. Langport, Portcullis.

Read, B. (2008) *Hooked-Clasps and Eyes: a Classification and Catalogue of Sharp- or Blunt-Hooked Clasps & Miscellaneous Objects with Hooks, Eyes, Loops, Rings or Toggles*. Langport, Portcullis.

Reed, M., ed. (1981) *The Ipswich Probate Inventories 1583-1631*. Woodbridge, Boydell Press for the Suffolk Records Society.

Robbins, K. (2012) *From Past to Present: Understanding the Impact of Sampling Bias on Data Recorded by the Portable Antiquities Scheme.* Unpublished PhD thesis, University of Southampton.

Shirley, E. P. (1869) An inventory of the effects of Henry Howard, K. G., Earl of Northampton, taken on his death in 1614, together with a transcript of his will. *Archaeologica* 42(2), 347–78.

Starkey, D., ed. (1998) *The Inventory of King Henry VIII. Society of Antiquaries MS 129 and British Library MS Harley 1419. Volume I: The Transcript.* London, Harvey Miller Publishers for Society of Antiquaries London.

Veblen, T. (1899) *The Theory of the Leisure Class.* New York.

'Wardens' Accounts and Court Minutes', *Goldsmiths' Company. K-L. 1566-7.ELIZ to 1573-14.ELIZ.*, vol. 9. London, Goldsmiths' Company Library.

Chapter 9

Cultural presumptions and curatorial context: reassessing the 'highland brooch' of Early Modern Scotland

Stuart Campbell

This chapter will discuss one of the most distinct objects of Early Modern dress in Britain and Ireland, an object which represents an apparently regional style in an age of commercial production and European-wide trends in dress. The highland brooch is an object which has attracted interest from the very beginning of antiquarianism and museums, and is an object that has defined Gaelic culture as both distinct and conservative in nature.

Yet for an object that was collected by antiquarians when it was almost still in use, its appearance in the literature is sporadic; no major article has considered it and modern work has in itself been limited by the lack of such major groundwork. It is an object type that has the unusual position of having an assured place in museum collections yet about which almost nothing is known, and this chapter will argue that its significance and very familiarity are built upon misperception and assumption. As well as this particularly Scottish context this object has a certain European interest. At a time when the dress accessories of western Europe acquired an apparent homogeneity from London to Nuremberg, the highland brooch stands out as a type that remained unique and distinct from these wider influences. Again, this distinction may be illusory rather than actual, but no less interesting for that.

The brooch itself is a simple object; a stout ring of metal (usually copper alloy) through which the cloth is pulled and held by a swivelling pin, the weight of cloth pulling the pin end fast against the body of the brooch. The type will be familiar to anyone who has studied the medieval period, or indeed earlier and has often (though never explicitly) been seen as a direct descendant of the medieval annular brooch, as a type which has lingered on in an area untouched by the progress of mainstream European life when it had fallen from use elsewhere in Europe. In the traditional interpretation, and these scant references will be discussed below, these brooches were used to fasten female clothing at the breast or neck in an identical fashion to the medieval annular brooches used across Europe some centuries before. They are distinct from the similar medieval types in being both larger and also decorated with elaborate engraving depicting stylised and fantastical animals and interlace and knotwork, representing a particular highland tradition (Fig. 9.1). It is clear from the numbers which survive (and from the excavated examples) that these brooches must have been numerous, in a variety of forms, across all social classes. Yet direct evidence for their use is sparse; one description comes in an unwittingly anachronistic projection of Early Modern dress backwards to the Medieval period

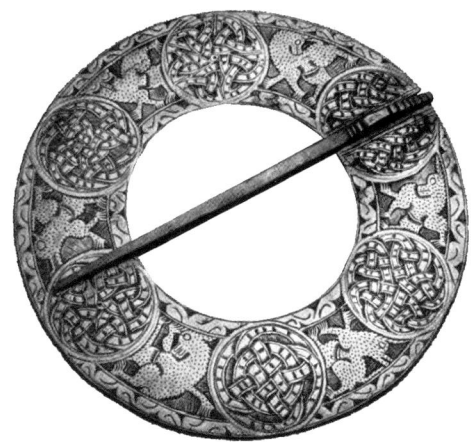

Fig. 9.1: This brass brooch from Tomintoul in the eastern highlands is typical of examples in museum collections and is seen as the characteristic type. Collections of National Museums Scotland (©National Museums Scotland).

where a seventeenth-century account of medieval deception has a man donning the disguise of a woman to meet with Robert II; his garb is a 'woman's habit, and a great brooch at his breast' (Marshall and Dalgleish 1991, 57). A more detailed description can be found in the journal of the traveller Martin Martin who in the 1690s described the fastening of the female plaid by brooches and buckles of brass or silver 'as broad as any plate' and 'curiously engraven with various animals' (Martin 1716, 209). These descriptions fit comfortably with the surviving brooches in museum collections, and many of these brooches can be ascribed seventeenth-century dates, partly on stylistic grounds as well by comparison with these few direct observations of these items in use. There appears to be only one depiction of such a brooch actually being worn, that of the painting popularly known as *The Hen Wife of Castle Grant,* painted in 1706 (now in the collections of the Scottish National Portrait Gallery), which depicts an elderly household servant using a brass brooch of this type to fasten the clothing at the throat of the sitter. An example which provides a very precise date is a brass brooch recovered from the wreck of HMS *Dartmouth* which foundered off Mull in 1695 (Martin 1998, 73–6). It is largely identical to that from Tomintoul shown in Figure 9.1 and, given the area of operations of the vessel, it is most likely to have come aboard from a west coast or Hebridean location. As will be discussed, this find-spot has some implications for the commonly presumed distribution of such brooches.

Valuable as these sources are their exactness also have disadvantages; there is a temptation perhaps to ascribe any brooch which fits these descriptions a seventeenth-century date, and as we will see below, this can create a problematic gap with other examples and types. It would be accurate to say that these brooches were worn during the seventeenth century in the Scottish highlands, but also very difficult to progress beyond that simple statement of fact. This difficulty is exacerbated, particularly as the canonical examples of the type are not those found by excavation, but rather those which have been bequeathed to museums from the eighteenth and nineteenth century onwards, and often with a disturbing lack of context or provenance. The most substantial collections of the type are housed in Inverness Museums, National Museums Scotland (henceforth NMS), and Aberdeen University Museums, and these large brass brooches have been seen as typical of the eastern highlands. It is a useful indication of the lack of published sources on these brooches that at this point the author is unable to back this assertion up with a published source; instead, it is an observation commonly expressed by curators at these same institutions and by itself an interesting example of the institutional culture and preconceptions that this article will address. Recent finds (to be discussed below) suggest this eastern distribution is not quite correct, and this may hinge on a single and simple fact; that the largest collections of these brooches are held by museums on the east coast of Scotland. While it may be reasonably observed that since its eighteenth-century foundation NMS has collected from the whole of Scotland (and should not be susceptible to such a bias) those brooches in the national collections suffer from another antiquarian curse; almost without exception they lack any find-spot information. Those few that do all have a find-spot in the eastern highlands, suggesting they may reflect the collecting bias of particular antiquarians or collectors.

What is then central to this chapter is one of the perils of museum curatorship, that it is all too common that collections are judged and curated on the assumptions which have been handed down by predecessors. Anyone who has worked in a museum or studied their collections will be all too aware how lacking in provenance or pedigree many significant collections are. To the archaeologist this may often take the form of objects (often by the drawerful) lacking find-spot information. To other researchers it may manifest in the form of a vague misapprehension about the subtle pull exerted by the prejudices and tastes of their antiquarian forebears in assembling a collection. In the case of the highland brooch, from their antiquarian inceptions Scottish museums have assiduously hoarded and acquired these brooches yet little appears to be known about their use or provenance. Their function and cultural significance appear to have been taken for granted. The first systematic representation of these brooches was in the work of the artist and antiquarian James Drummond, then the curator of the Scottish National Gallery and who specialised in highly detailed colour depictions of antiquities and archaeological sites. Tellingly, Drummond's work was published after his death as part of a larger work, 'Ancient Scottish Weapons' (Drummond and Anderson 1881), where these brooches appear alongside sporrans, targes, powder horns and Lochaber axes as the familiar embodiments of an alien and warlike Gaelic culture, yet one whose strangeness had been made utterly familiar in the British popular imagination. This wider repackaging (or indeed, outright fabrication) of a Scottish highland culture has been thoroughly covered elsewhere with antiquarians, fantasists and popular writers producing a reimagining of highland culture from the eighteenth century onwards that that was presented, often with a wilful blindness, as an ancient cultural tradition (Trevor-Roper 1983). Drummond had recorded these objects when, like the targes and sporrans, they were an utterly familiar part of a Gaelic culture which had been assimilated into Victorian society; by the late eighteenth century these brooches were being produced by urban silversmiths and they gradually became incorporated into the 'Highland dress' which was the synthetic product of an increasingly urban and lowland Scotland (Marshall and Dalgleish 1991, 62–5). Yet most striking is the manner in which the synthetic Gaelic past influenced both popular culture and antiquarian pursuits. In 1851 Daniel Wilson considered the material culture of the early modern highlands as the manifestation of an ancient tradition that was terminated in the 'last fatal struggle of the clans on Culloden moor' (Wilson 1851, 220). In hindsight it seems reasonable to argue that the interest antiquarians displayed in these objects was as much a product of this assumed importance rather than an objective appreciation of what they were. In the case of the NMS collections this can be seen in the way these brooches were catalogued and the other material with which they were associated. Both highland brooches and the medieval annular types were subsumed (alongside any peculiar or unusual type) within a category defined as 'brooches with old style pins', which still exists today within the museum database. It would be unfair to criticise nineteenth-century curators from a modern perspective, but this does suggest a lack of critical curiosity regarding the artefacts in question. With both this lack of critical interest and the lack of concern for cultural authenticity it is perhaps not surprising that that many iconic brooches held within the national collections have proven to be nineteenth-century replicas (Caldwell et al. 2002).

To the Victorian curator then, these brooches fitted comfortably into a pre-ordained cultural niche, yet the culturally distinct, conservative and independent highland culture which apparently produced these objects is very much a fiction of nineteenth-century Romanticism. Many of these brooches, though unique and rare beasts from a European perspective, reference also the sentiments, purpose and aesthetics of that jewellery which can be comfortably accommodated within the European tradition. It is also the case that the collections of Scottish museums suffer perhaps more than most from objects loaded with past assumptions about their significance. In recent years NMS curators have usefully revisited many apparently canonical finds such as the Bute Mazer (Caldwell and Dalgleish 2012) and the Monymusk Reliquary (Caldwell 2001) and reappraised their significance. This is a crucial point; it is essential for institutions to reassess significant objects whose acquisitions have often taken place uncritically or unquestioningly. The aim of this chapter is not to criticise past or recent publications and interpretations but rather to observe how difficult it can be to work with objects which lack context both in terms of simple provenance and also in terms of the rationale behind their acquisition.

When considering how museum collections are created over time it is clear also that then, as now, there can be significant scholarly and curatorial biases which can affect the assessment of an object. Some of these biases may be less evident to historians of costume or art historians, but to the archaeologist the definition and interpretation of museum collections can often, like St Peter at the gates, seem a capricious yet predictable judgment; it is often the case that objects made of precious metal and of a certain quality are promoted to the fine arts while those of base metal or poor workmanship are consigned to archaeology or folk culture. A case in point can be found in the NMS catalogue of medieval and early modern objects (Glenn 2003) where the precious metal examples of highland brooches are categorised as 'Gothic' and discussed in isolation from the both base metal examples and silver examples of lesser quality and execution. The conventional view of these brass brooches has been discussed above, and can be contrasted by the pull in another direction regarding the second type of brooch to be considered in detail here.

The collections at NMS include a small and apparently distinct group of silver annular brooches, of either circular or octagonal form, which frequently include inscriptions in black letter script, the sharply linear and angular script that was used on jewellery and other items from the later fourteenth century onwards. An example of this type can be seen in Figure 9.2; found in Kengharair on Mull, and made from

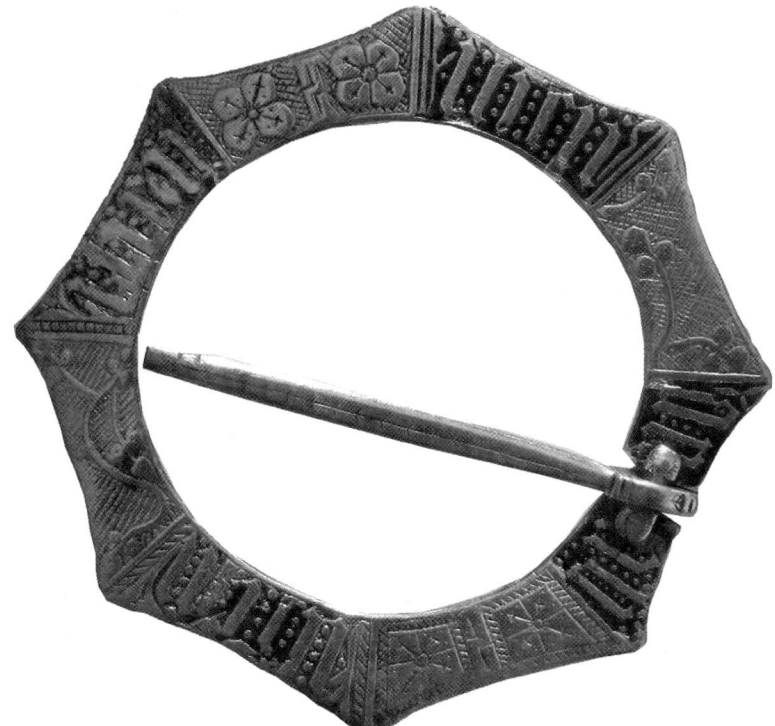

Fig. 9.2: Silver and niello brooch from Kengharair on the Isle of Mull. Collections of National Museums Scotland (©National Museums Scotland).

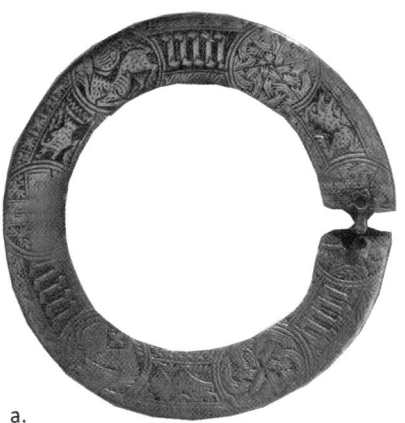
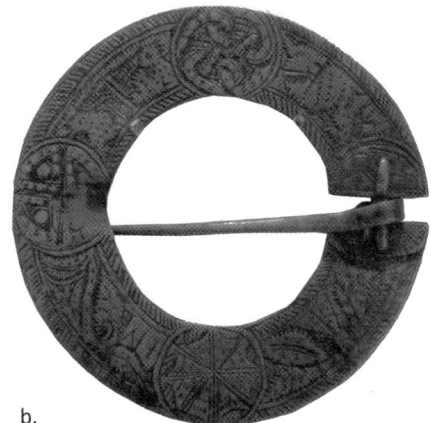

Fig. 9.3: a. Silver and niello brooch from Ballachulish; b. brass example from the eastern highlands. Collections of National Museums Scotland (©Crown Office).

sheet silver, the brooch is heavily decorated with both letters and various symbols and motifs picked out in niello. One side has the inscription 'IHCN' and 'ANAN' (for *Ihesus nazarenus*) interspersed with motifs of foliage and flowers whilst the other side has a series of zoomorphic animals (Glenn 2003, 72–3). These are a visually striking class of objects and the use of black letter is an assurance of date *c.* 1500. Another example was found near Ballachulish, and is substantially similar, being decorated with an illegible Black letter inscription interspersed with knotwork and a variety of wild and otherwise fantastical beasts (Fig. 9.3). A third example is known only from its publication in the late nineteenth century; of similarly octagonal form, and decorated in an identical manner, the only provenance is that it was in the possession of the (then late) Lord Bellahouston, its current whereabouts is unknown (Brook 1889).

Conventionally the find-spots of these brooches have meant they have been ascribed to a distinct West Highland culture, and in standard works they are considered as part of a larger West Highland tradition of silver working which includes such remarkable pieces as the Glenlyon and Ballochyle brooches (in the collections of the British Museum and NMS respectively), substantial and elaborate silver gilt brooches often set with gems and rock crystal and imbued – through either inscriptions or materials – with talismanic or healing properties (though it must be stressed also that a silvermsith's mark suggests that the Ballochyle brooch was made in a lowland burgh) (Marshall and Dalgleish 1991, 56–9). Along with such distinctive items as the Guthrie bell shrine these brooches have been seen as representative of a maritime Gàidhealtachd which stretched from Argyll to the Hebrides (National Museum of Antiquities of Scotland 1982, 58–60). There is no doubt that some of this material culture has a distinct West Highland heritage, to consider the Ballochyle brooch and the Guthrie bell shrine, for example, is to consider the material evidence of a truly distinct culture, and one with connections both across the Irish sea and further afield. It is the case also that the

Mull and Ballachulish brooches undoubtedly share some traits with these other types; all for example have similar religious or talismanic inscriptions. Yet these high status and elaborate examples stand apart for what they are, symbols both of magical power and worldly status which were worn by the heads of great families; the rather more modest silver and niello examples hardly compare. This comparison relies also on a hierarchical interpretation, and one arguably typical of an art historical position: that the lower quality objects must be copying the high quality examples rather than, for example, all such brooches referencing the same cultural tradition.

Yet find-spot aside, it is reasonable to question to what extent these silver and neillo brooches are part of a West Highland culture or represent something wholly different. While naturally the focus of museum displays and exhibition catalogues have been on the silver types they are somewhat outnumbered by brass examples of the type, including ones from excavations at Castle Sween and Achanduin Castle in Argyll and seven others in the collections of the National Museums Scotland (Caldwell 1996, 546). The Mull and Ballachulish examples are in no way representative of the type, but the happenstance of their production in silver has determined their transformation into *objects d'art*, coming to represent the type as a whole and ensuring they are compared with other silver objects from the western highlands rather than more suitable, yet more humble types.

Superficially, on art historical grounds and by dint of distributions of examples found in museums collections these brooches appear as two distinct classes of objects, one confined to each coast of Scotland. By contrast, it is clear that the biases of museum collections and the tendency to distinguish between fine art and archaeology have teased apart a coherent group of objects into two distinct groups. This assertion can be proved very simply; compare the Ballachulish brooch to an example from the eastern highlands and it is clear that both are largely identical (Fig. 9.3). While it is made of brass, the eastern example is of the same size, appearance and has the same knotwork roundels and zoomorphic decoration. A crucial difference is that the example from the eastern highlands lacks a black letter inscription, which are undoubtedly more common on western examples. Nevertheless, as will be argued below, the use of black letter can be interpreted as something more than a regional style. Both also share what is a feature of all these brooches, the unusual pin head, the details of which can be seen in Figure 9.4 (see below). Although conventional interpretation would separate them by at least a century and 150 miles they are in effect different examples of the same object. Curatorial assumptions have shepherded these brooches into a distinct group of seventeenth-century date and made of brass with a distribution in the eastern highlands, while creating another group of fifteenth- to sixteenth-century date, made of silver with a western distribution, yet it can be demonstrated there is no real difference between these two types, and that their essential features overlap both chronologically and stylistically.

Thus far, the examples which have been discussed have almost all been those from museum collections, or those chance finds which compare with them in

9. Cultural presumptions and curatorial context 177

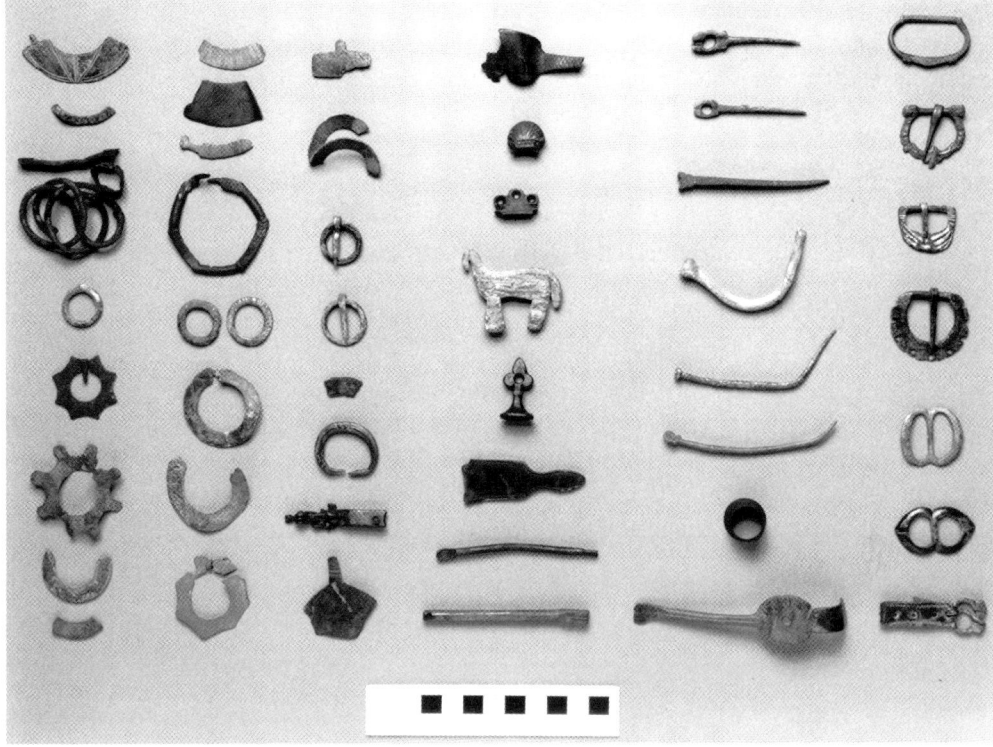

Fig. 9.4: Assemblages from burgh and urban sites show that these brooches were used alongside a wide range of mainstream European dress accessories and other items. Collections of Inverness Museum & Art Gallery (©Crown Office).

quality and workmanship. Yet this in itself introduces a bias: they are all objects whose quality has ensured that they are kept and donated to institutions. In the case of the brooches from Castle Sween and Achanduin Castle (discussed above) it can be seen how the introduction of excavated examples can quickly change the context and interpretation of large groups of material. As well as relying on these scant historical references and brooches in museum collections this article will rely on material from excavations carried out at a number of key sites as well as chance finds made in recent years. In this sense it is demonstrative also how interdependent the work of archaeologists, art historians and costume historians can be and the author would argue that the greatest potential for interpreting these brooches is by consideration of excavated material. However iconic many of these well known brooches are, and however firmly bedded in the post-medieval era they are still floating free of archaeological and cultural context regarding both use and antecedent. In examining the wide range of these brooches that have been found by excavation and metal detector users in recent years it is clear that those examples in museums are a small and unrepresentative sample, and that these brooches existed in a wide variety of forms and types which vary greatly in terms of quality. This in turn suggests that such brooches were used and had meaning across a wide range of social classes beyond what might be suggested by the opulent and elaborate brooches that are usually used to illustrate the type.

The brooches recovered from a series of excavations or reappraisals of key sites on both the East and West Highlands provide an opportunity to provide a clear context and antecedents for a class of object which otherwise hovers mysteriously between the medieval and post-medieval periods. They demonstrate also that the suggested distributions for the various types of brooch differ markedly from those suggested by museum collections. For example while a copper-alloy octagonal brooch from Carrick Castle in Argyll (Ewart and Baker 1998, 962) may be superficially similar to the form and appearance of the Mull and Bellahouston brooches it can also be directly compared to several types from the east coast of Scotland, including two examples from Urquhart Castle (Samson 1982, 573). In fact, however unusual the octagonal shape of the brooch might appear to be, it has proven to be an extremely common type amongst the metal detected finds made around east coast highland burghs like Cromarty,[1] Fortrose[2] and Dornoch[3] where a number have been recovered, all made from copper alloy. The number of brooches which have been discovered in this manner is surprising, and like those from excavations, they are often cheaply and simply made, although otherwise sharing their essential features with the larger and more elaborate examples.

In recent years a number of the distinctive large brass brooches have been found on the west coast. To the brooch from the Dartmouth can be added recent discoveries including an intact brooch from Ulva,[4] one from near Fort William[5] and a pin from Bostadh, Isle of Lewis.[6] The brooch from Ulva is of particular interest as on the rear face it is decorated with two small crosses which, by comparison with other examples, suggests strongly that it was given as a betrothal present (Caldwell 1998).

This symmetry of distribution that these chance finds suggest can be seen among many other excavated finds. A distinctive style from Dunstaffnage Castle in Argyll (Lewis 1996, 583) can also be given an eastern parallel in an example from Kildrummy Castle in Aberdeenshire (Apted 1963, 49); the decoration set at right angles clearly follows the same design as the four large roundels set every 90° on the more elaborate examples and large numbers of this type have again been found as metal detector finds in east coast sites such as Dornoch (Fig. 9.4). The ubiquity of the brooches raises an interesting question; while it has conventionally been the case that these brooches have been considered from the top down, the high quality examples that survived in Victorian museum collections were very much in the minority in the society that used them. The evidence of both excavated sites and metal detectorist finds demonstrates that these were objects that were used widely throughout society. However unusual the octagonal form may appear when seen in the isolation of the Mull and Ballochyle examples it is clear that it must have been common throughout society; many of the Dornoch examples are cheaply made from thin sheet metal.

While it might seem natural to see the larger and ornate examples as at the top of a hierarchy it is clear that they instead are elaborate and sophisticated versions of these everyday examples, and a simple copper-alloy version of the knopped octagonal form of the Bellahouston and Ballochyle brooches can be seen in the left in Figure 9.4. Rather than these high status examples serving as the influence for lower status examples, it is clear that the Ballochyle and Glenlyon brooches have evolved from a variety of simple forms. What this may indicate is the importance of this type of brooch in highland society, an object which was in use throughout the social order.

Many of these simpler brooches share design features with the earlier medieval types; the octagonal brooch from Urquhart Castle has features that can both be paralleled on the medieval brooches of the fourteenth century and on those later brooches of the sixteenth century. The unusual octagonal shape of these brooches can in itself be traced back to a variation of standard medieval annular brooch found in Scotland (Glenn 3003, 75). Overall then, the excavated evidence would indicate that when the rest of the British Isles (and indeed Europe) had stopped using such brooches by c. 1400 (Egan and Forsyth 1997, 220) these objects continued in use in much of Scotland. To the antiquarian, and indeed the early twentieth-century archaeologist, this could be explained easily; the highlands represented a conservative and backward culture (Curwen 1938). Yet this explanation hardly stands scrutiny when we consider that the same culture that used these brooches could not be said to be backward or lacking in cultural means or fiscal power. Notwithstanding the power and influence of the Lordship of the Isles, those other brooches come from sites of the secular elites, and the assemblage at Castle Urquhart for example, contains also a fragment of black letter metal from a bowl or mazer, an object which again would be at home in a wider British or European context (Samson 1982, 474). Yet this item of domestic metalwork shares the same lettering with brooches which, again by these wider standards, would seem profoundly strange and foreign.

However unusual these brooches might appear, this use of black letter inscriptions, more than a simple dating tool, suggests instead that the makers and wearers of these brooches were familiar with European social mores and religious beliefs. The use of black letter became common on European jewellery from the mid-fourteenth century onwards, and the highland brooches follow this same style; like other European jewellery the inscriptions often reference playful or romantic sentiments and were clearly given as betrothal gifts. This is most obvious in the large brooch recovered from Kindrochit Castle in Aberdeenshire and its use of the amorous French sentiment 'friend of my heart' in again, a black letter inscription surrounded by floral motifs (Glenn 2003, 68–9). The use of jewellery to make a romantic statement is one familiar from early modern Europe and the significance of this for highland brooches will be discussed in detail later. The other recurring ideas and sentiment in the brooch inscriptions also closely follows a major trend in European religious belief which is again widely reflected in jewellery and personal adornment. The repeated use of religious inscription on Scottish examples has often been assumed to refer backwards to the common medieval apotropaic device of '*ihesus nazarenus rex ioderoum*' (Lightbown 1992, 99), again perhaps an assumption that these are items which are the product of a conservative culture. However the legend 'IHCN NA' used on the Mull brooch refers instead to the Cult of the Holy Name, a devotion which became which became increasingly popular throughout Europe from the fifteenth century, the time when these brooches were produced. The most visible personal symbol of this devotion was an object thus marked, which may be a dress accessory or an item of personal jewellery (Blake *et al.* 2003). In this European context, however strange these brooches might appear, the same lettering can be paralleled on a wide variety of personal objects such as jewellery and dress accessories.

Other examples also demonstrate this wider engagement with European styles: a silver brooch from Rannoch Moor shows a distinct Renaissance influence in the choice of motifs which nestle between the otherwise typical knotwork of the designs (National Museums Scotland, accession number H.NGA 260). The use of the floral and vegetal design on the Mull brooch is also noteworthy. The use of flowers and floral sprays is a constant with romantic jewellery of the fifteenth century (Campbell 2009, 94) and with their use of black letter and floral decoration, the Mull and Kindrochit brooches could reasonably be compared, in style and influence, if not in form, to the amorous jewellery which comprises the heart of the Fishpool Hoard (Cherry 1973).

The question should not be so much why an apparently archaic form survived, but rather why it incorporated and referenced mainstream European cultural references, religious beliefs and jewellery styles, all the while retaining the same unchanging form. This suggests not so much a culture which was cut off from mainstream beliefs, or one that rejected innovation through cultural conservatism, but rather one to which the function that these brooches played and the meanings that they had were highly important. In other words, the cultural and intellectual sentiments of mainstream European thought were adapted to a particular class of object rather than having a wider influence on tastes and fashions. It should be stressed at this point that the modern finds support the interpretation as a highland type, that is, they all have been found in the area of Scotland which in both cultural and political terms would have formed a distinct entity at the time these brooches were in use.

This coherence in both object type and distribution suggests that these brooches had a distinct cultural meaning, and any interpretation must be rooted in a wider framework that considers the social role that they must have played. These objects represent both an individual choice while at the same time reflecting a group identity; they are a blend of social, economic and cultural considerations (Fisher and Loren 2003). It can be argued that archaeology represents the best chance of recovering and analysing the cultural experiences of groups that depart from what might be categorised as wider cultural norms (White 2013, 58). In this particular case, these brooches could be said to bridge this often challenging interpretative gap between individual choice and the norms of the society, representing as they do the creative act of an individual that in turn references wider social norms.

The act of the individual is best discerned by the highly unusual features of the brooches themselves for it is clear that in their methods of manufacture they differ markedly from the techniques that might be expected from a skilled metalworker. Almost without exception they lack evidence of access to any specialist equipment or skills and all examples are not cast but made from sheet metal, sometimes roughly cut or reshaped with some evidence of recycling existing objects. Where the two ends of the metal meet at the pin rebate there is no evidence of brazing, but rather sometimes the two ends are clipped or riveted together, sometimes simply held together by the constriction of the pin. Overall, these brooches demonstrate a lack of the skills and techniques that would have been common to any metalworker of the period, and a lack of access to equipment that would have been common in any workshop. Where additional decorative techniques are used they are almost wholly restricted to niello, which compared to enamelling or gilding, is a technique that requires only commonly sourced materials and has a melting point below that of any furnace. Overall, the skill of engraving varies widely also and overall they do not appear to be the product of a skilled craftsman. They appear to have been made by a diversity of individuals who varied greatly in the skills and tools that they possessed.

This observation tallies well with an observation made by travellers in the region at the end of the period at which these brooches were in use, both Martin Martin and (rather later) John Lane Buchanan comment on the tendency for highland males to make such objects as buckles and brooches, with the latter commenting 'that the common people are wondrously ingenious. They make hooks for fishing, cast metal buckles, brooches and rings for their favourite females' (Brook 1889, 197).

The evidence of the brooches themselves suggest that Martin and Buchanan were recording the last vestiges of a much older tradition of gift giving and jewellery making and the brooches discussed here would accord easily with these accounts. Many, as the quotes above imply, were given for romantic reasons, and evidence for this varies from the clear amatory intent of the inscription on the Kindrochit brooch to the decoration on the back of the example from Ulva which again implies a marriage gift or similar. The same cultural behaviour can be seen also in other, similar objects, including the silver heart shaped brooches which appear to have been in use from the early eighteenth century and which were given both as romantic gifts and as protective amulets and which were particularly popular in the highlands (Marshall and Dalgleish 1991, 41).

The cultural importance of this practice can be gauged by its popularity, traversing a maritime Gaelic culture that was increasingly hostile against central authority to a relatively urban and increasingly English-speaking highland culture in the east. While it may be tempting to view the longevity of these brooches as illustrating a conservative culture there are many reasons instead that we should view it as assertive and confident practice. These areas are not those which are rural or remote, for while the practice of home-made objects could be conceived of in some remote communities it is clear that these brooches were made and used also in well connected elite sites such as castles as well as the burghs of the east coast. The burghs were the legally franchised core of Scottish society; they functioned as both political and economic hubs and were one of the defining features of early modern Scotland. Yet in the highland burghs it is clear that these brooches were made and used alongside a variety of other, more cosmopolitan objects. The assemblage in Figure 9.4 includes, for example, a seal matrix of seventeenth-century form, a variety of buckles of standard European sixteenth- to seventeenth-century types and imported knives of the same period from Germany and the Low Countries. In this context it is clear these brooches functioned alongside what would be recognised as the material culture of any early modern European urban settlement. The equivalent dress accessories that could have succeeded these brooches would clearly have been available, but we can presume that the local population chose not to use them as they lacked the cultural significance and social meaning of these brooches.

This fact by itself suggests how fatally flawed the category of folk history or folk jewellery (the latter a favourite terminology in museum catalogues) can be; in this case folk culture was clearly part of an urban culture and its makers and users presumably saw no distinction between what would appear to the modern researcher as two different, and sometimes competing, strands. The material evidence of access to imported goods indicates also that this tradition is of more than Scottish or British interest; however vernacular this custom may appear, it can be paralleled in other parts of Europe. In Estonia a very similar cultural tradition can be identified, where the annular brooches of the medieval period continued in use after the fifteenth century and evolved in the post-medieval period into large and elaborate items used as part of traditional dress (Kirme 2002). In Estonia these brooches had both symbolic and practical functions, the latter most notably in that they were necessary to secure the complex and multi-layered female clothing at the neck. This may be analogous for Scotland also, since the point at which these brooches developed and continued in use was the point also at which it is generally accepted the Scottish Highlands developed its own highly distinctive regional dress (Trevor-Roper 1983, 18–20). Indeed, the accounts of such objects in use that were quoted earlier show such brooches being used with what may loosely be termed a 'highland dress'. While this should not be ignored, it is also true that these brooches were in use in areas in the eastern highlands where it can be confidently said clothes would have resembled much lowland (and indeed, European) garb. Nevertheless this is a reminder that these objects should not be viewed as purely archaeological finds, divorced from the clothing that they were an integral part of. A useful comparison to both Estonia and Scotland can be found in recent work on dress in Early Modern Hungary, demonstrating again how mainstream European objects can be assimilated and adapted into regional cultures and clothing styles (Mérai 2010).

Within this wider European context, rather than defining these objects as belonging to folk culture it might be more helpful to recognise them as representing very dynamic practices, where object types are retained or accepted because they serve a highly specific purpose in that culture. These, as we have seen with highland brooches, often reflect a reinterpretation of mainstream cultural ideas in a profoundly local setting, something reinforced by both an art historical consideration of these brooches and their archaeological contexts. This chapter has perhaps only touched slightly on what is a long lived and complex tradition of one particular object type, and as much as it serves as any illustration of an object type it perhaps more of a cautionary tale, showing how easily objects can be taken for granted, and how the same objects can mean entirely different things to different disciplines. What this illustrates is how interdependent and intertwined the work of archaeologists, curators and costume historians actually is, and how judgments made in one discipline can have effects and unlooked for consequences in a wholly different field of study.

Notes

1. Allocated to Cromarty Museum, reference number TT.118/07.
2. Allocated to Groan House Museum, reference number TT.18/04.
3. Allocated to Inverness Museum & Art Gallery with reference number TT.153/97.
4. Allocated to Argyll & Bute Museums service with reference number TT.07/98.
5. Allocated to Inverness Museum & Art Gallery with reference number TT.83/06.
6. Allocated to Western Isles Museums service with reference number TT.15/04.

Bibliography

Apted, M. R. (1963) Excavation at Kildrummy Castle, Aberdeenshire, 1952–62. *Proceedings of the Society of Antiquaries of Scotland* 96, 208–36.

Blake, H., Egan, G., Hurst, J., and New, E. (2003) From popular devotion to resistance and revival in England: the cult of the Holy Name of Jesus and the Reformation. In D. Gaimster and R. Gilchrist (eds.) *The Archaeology of Reformation, 1480-1580*, 176–202. Leeds, Maney (Society for Post-Medieval Archaeology Monograph 1).

Brook, A. J. S. (1889) Notice of a silver brooch with black letter inscription and ornamentation in niello, the property of Miss Steven of Bellahouston, and of a large brass highland brooch with incised ornamentation, the property of Mrs W R Mitford, 33 Coates Gardens, Edinburgh. *Proceedings of the Society of Antiquaries of Scotland* 23, 192–9.

Caldwell, D. H. (1996) Other artefacts from Castle Sween. In G. Ewart and J. Triscott Archaeological excavations at Castle Sween, Knapdale, Argyll & Bute, 1989–90. *Proceedings of the Society of Antiquaries of Scotland* 126, 517–57.

Caldwell, D. H. (1998) Unpublished NMAS report on Treasure Trove case TT.07/98. Held in Treasure Trove Unit archives, National Museums Scotland.

Caldwell, D. H. (2001) The Monymusk reliquary: the Breccbennach of St Columba? *Proceedings of the Society of Antiquaries of Scotland* 131, 267–82.

Caldwell, D. H., Eremin, K., Moran, J., Tate, J. and Wilthew, P. (2002) Highland brooches. *Antique Metalware Society Journal* 10, 33–9.

Caldwell, D. H. and Dalgleish, G. (2012) The Bute or Bannatyne Mazer – two different vessels. In A. Ritchie (ed.) *Historic Bute: Land and People*. Edinburgh, Scottish Society for Northern Studies.

Campbell, M. (2009) *Medieval Jewellery in Europe 1100-1500*. London, V&A.

Cherry, J. (1973) VII. The Medieval Jewellery from the Fishpool, Nottinghamshire, Hoard. *Archaeologia (Second Series)* 104(1), 307–21.

Curwen, E. (1938) The Hebrides: a cultural backwater. *Antiquity* 12(47), 261–89.
Drummond, J. and Anderson, J. (1881) *Ancient Scottish Weapons: a Series of Drawings*. Edinburgh, Waterston.
Egan, G. and Forsyth, H. (1997) Wound wire and silver gilt: changing fashions in dress accessories c. 1400–c. 1600. In D. R. Gaimster and P. Stamper (eds.) *The Age of Transition: the Archaeology of English Culture 1400-1600*, 215–38. Oxford, Oxbow Books.
Ewart, G. and Baker, F. (1998) Carrick Castle: symbol and source of Campbell power in south Argyll from the 14th to the 17th century. *Proceedings of the Society of Antiquaries of Scotland*, 128, 937–1016.
Fisher, G. and Loren, D. (2003) Embodying identity in archaeology. *Cambridge Archaeological Journal* 13, 225–30.
Glenn, V. (2003) *Romanesque and Gothic: Decorative Metalwork and Ivory Carvings in the Museum of Scotland*. Edinburgh, National Museums of Scotland.
Kirme, K. (2002) *Eesti rahvapärased ehted: 13. sajand-20. sajandi algus*. Talin, Eesti Entsüklopeediakirjastus.
Lewis, J. (1996) Dunstaffnage Castle, Argyll & Bute: excavations in the north tower and east range, 1987–94. *Proceedings of the Society of Antiquaries of Scotland* 126, 559–603.
Lightbown, R. W. (1992) *Medieval European Jewellery*. London, Victoria and Albert Museum.
Marshall, R. K. and Dalgleish, G. (1991) *The Art of Jewellery in Scotland*. Edinburgh, HMSO.
Martin, M. (1716) *A Description of the Western Islands of Scotland: Containing a Full Account of Their Situation* (abbreviated title). London, printed for printed for A. Bell; T. Varnam and J. Osborn; W. Taylor and J. Baker and T. Warner.
Martin, C. (1998) *Scotland's Historic Shipwrecks*. London, Batsford.
Mérai, D. (2010) *"The True and Exact Dresses and Fashion": Archaeological Clothing Remains and their Social Contexts in Sixteenth- and Seventeenth-Century Hungary*. Oxford, Archaeopress (British Archaeological Reports, International Series 2078).
National Museum of Antiquities of Scotland (1982). *Angels, Nobles and Unicorns: Art and Patronage in Medieval Scotland; a Handbook Published in Connection with an Exhibition Held at the National Museum of Scotland, August 12-September 26, 1982*. Edinburgh, National Museum of Antiquities of Scotland.
Samson, R. (1982) Finds from Urquhart Castle in the National Museum, Edinburgh. *Proceedings of the Society of Antiquaries of Scotland* 112, 465–76).
Trevor-Roper, H. (1983) The invention of tradition: the highland tradition of Scotland. In E. Hobsbawm and T. Ranger (eds.) *The Invention of Tradition*, 15–42. Cambridge, Cambridge University Press.
White, C. L. (2013) Trans-Atlantic perspectives on eighteenth-century clothing. In J. Symonds, A. Badcock and J. Oliver (eds.) *Historical Archaeologies of Cognition: Explorations into Faith, Hope and Charity*, 57–71. Sheffield, Equinox.
Wilson, D. (1851) *The Archaeology and Prehistoric Annals of Scotland*. Edinburgh, Sutherland & Knox.